HOW TO PLAY PICKLEBALL: FROM BEGINNER TO BRILLIANT

Learn the Rules, Techniques and Strategies to Master the Game

Sam Alexander

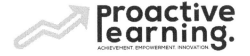

proactive
learning.

ACHIEVEMENT. EMPOWERMENT. INNOVATION.

HOW TO PLAY PICKLEBALL: FROM BEGINNER TO BRILLIANT
Learn the Rules, Techniques and Strategies to Master the Game

Publisher's Note:

Although every precaution has been taken to ensure that the information in this book was correct at the time of publication, the author and publisher do not assume and hereby disclaim any liability to any party for any loss, damage, or disruption caused by errors or omissions, whether such errors or omissions result from negligence, accident, or any other causes.

The information contained in this book is intended to be educational and for informational purposes only. The author or publisher makes no representations or warranties with respect to the accuracy, fitness, or completeness of the information, text, graphics, images, links, and other items contained in this book. The book is not to serve as a substitute for personal professional instruction. All physical activities, including pickleball, carry the risk of injury or physical harm. Readers should seek professional advice before beginning any new exercise program. The author and the publisher are in no way liable for any misuse of the material or any injury or harm that may occur as a result of following the techniques and advice presented in this book.

ISBN: 978-0-6458961-0-7

TABLE OF CONTENTS

INTRODUCTION

WELCOME TO THE WORLD OF PICKLEBALL!

Welcome to the exciting world of pickleball, a sport that has taken the world by storm and captured the hearts of players of all ages and skill levels from around the globe. Pickleball, the unique paddle sport that fuses elements of tennis, badminton, and table tennis, has become a global phenomenon for several compelling reasons. What sets pickleball apart and fuels its passionate following is a combination of accessibility, addictive gameplay, and the sense of community it fosters.

Pickleball's widespread popularity is rooted in its accessibility, welcoming players of all ages and skill levels. With its modified court size, lower net height, and lightweight paddles, pickleball provides an inclusive platform for everyone to participate and enjoy the game. Whether you're a beginner or a seasoned athlete, pickleball embraces inclusivity and invites you to join in the fun. The simplicity of pickleball's rules and its quick learning curve make it accessible to newcomers, while its versatility allows experienced players to continuously refine their skills. Combining elements from different sports, such as tennis, badminton, and table tennis, pickleball offers a unique playing experience that is easy to learn yet challenging to master.

The addictive gameplay of pickleball keeps players engaged and yearning for more. Fast-paced rallies, strategic shot placement, and the thrill of executing well-timed smashes and finesse shots create an exciting and adrenaline-filled experience. Pickleball's dynamic gameplay offers a captivating playing experience that hooks players from the moment they step onto the court.

Pickleball's strong sense of community is another key aspect that contributes to its passionate following. The friendly and welcoming community of players embraces newcomers, fostering connections and creating lasting friendships. Pickleball communities, clubs, and tournaments provide opportunities for players to socialize, share experiences, and support one another both on and off the court. This sense of camaraderie adds to the enduring love for the sport.

In this book, we will delve deep into the world of pickleball, exploring its origins, rules, techniques, strategies, and the wealth of resources available to players. We will guide you on a journey of skill development, tactical insights, and expert advice, equipping you with the tools you need to excel on the pickleball court. Whether you're a seasoned athlete or a curious newcomer seeking a thrilling recreational activity, this book will provide everything you need to know about pickleball and why it has become one of the most exciting and engaging sports in the world today.

So, get ready to embark on a thrilling adventure that introduces you to the incredible sport of pickleball. Discover why it has become a global sensation, captivating the hearts and minds of players worldwide. Embrace the excitement, joy, and sense of belonging that pickleball offers. Welcome to the wonderful world of pickleball!

OVERVIEW OF THE BOOK'S CONTENTS

This book takes a comprehensive approach to pickleball, covering everything from the fundamentals to advanced techniques and strategies. It is designed to cater to players of all levels, from beginners to experienced players looking to elevate their game. Each chapter is carefully structured to provide a well-rounded understanding of the sport, focusing on different aspects of the game and providing practical tips and insights.

The book begins by establishing a strong foundation with chapters dedicated to the basics of pickleball, including an overview of the game, its history, and the benefits it offers. Readers will learn about court navigation, rules and scoring, and essential gear for optimal performance.

From there, the book progresses to more specific areas of the game, such as serving strategies, third shot tactics, and offensive and defensive play.

Throughout the book, detailed instructions and tips are provided to help players improve their skills and develop a competitive edge. The content is presented in a clear and concise manner, with easy-to-follow explanations and illustrations to enhance understanding. There are also **Fast facts** and **Top tips** included in each chapter, as well as **Drills** to hone your skills and perfect your performance.

Additionally, the book emphasizes the importance of technique, strategy, and sportsmanship, ensuring that readers not only become proficient players but also embody the spirit of the game.

Whether you are a novice or an experienced pickleball player, this book serves as a comprehensive guide to help you enhance your skills, gain a deeper understanding of the game, and maximize your enjoyment on the court. With its systematic approach and expert advice, it provides the tools and knowledge needed to take your pickleball game to the next level.

Fast facts:

Pickleball is the fastest-growing sport in America, with a staggering growth rate of 158.6% over the last three years and a current estimated growth rate of 10-15% annually. The number of players playing pickleball has nearly doubled in the seven years from 2014 to 2021, with 8.9 million players in the United States of America as of early 2023.

CHAPTER 1   THE FUNDAMENTALS OF PICKLEBALL

Chapter 1 sets the stage for your exciting journey into the world of this unique sport. In this chapter, we will explore the core elements that make pickleball so special and lay the foundation for your pickleball adventure.

First, we will answer the question on every newcomer's mind: What is pickleball? You will gain a clear understanding of this paddle sport, its rules, equipment, and gameplay. Discover how pickleball combines the best of tennis, badminton, and table tennis to create a thrilling experience on the court.

Next, we will delve into the rich history of pickleball. Uncover its humble beginnings and learn about the visionaries who shaped it into the global phenomenon it is today.

Pickleball isn't just a game; it offers numerous benefits for physical and mental well-being. We will explore these benefits, from improving fitness and coordination to fostering social connections.

Understanding the pickleball court is essential, so we will navigate its lines and zones, unraveling their purpose and how they contribute to gameplay.

Lastly, we will decode the rules and scoring system, ensuring you have a solid grasp of the game's mechanics.

Join us in Chapter 1 as we lay the groundwork for your pickleball journey. Whether you're an absolute beginner or a player with more experience, this chapter will equip you with the knowledge and insights you need to embark on this thrilling sport. Get ready to dive into the fundamentals of pickleball and experience the joy, strategy, and excitement that await you on the court!

1.1   WHAT IS PICKLEBALL?

In pickleball, players use specially designed paddles to hit a lightweight, perforated plastic ball over the net and into the opposing team's court. The objective is to execute well-placed shots that challenge the opponents and prevent them from returning the ball successfully. With its smaller court size and slower ball speed compared to tennis, pickleball emphasizes precision, agility, and quick reflexes. Players must employ strategic shot selection, adapt their footwork to swiftly maneuver around the court, and anticipate their opponents' moves to gain the upper hand.

One of the appealing aspects of pickleball is its versatility, as it can be played in both singles and doubles formats. Singles matches offer a more intense and focused gameplay experience, requiring players to rely solely on their own skills and tactics. Doubles matches, on the other hand, encourage teamwork, communication, and coordination between partners. This flexibility allows players to choose the format that suits their preferences and enables the sport to cater to a wide range of individuals.

The scoring system in pickleball follows a similar format to tennis, where players or teams aim to accumulate points by winning rallies. However, only the serving player or team can score points. The first player or team to reach 11 points, while leading by a margin of at least two points, wins the game. This scoring system ensures that matches remain competitive and provides opportunities for exciting comebacks.

So, whether you're a seasoned athlete looking to try a new sport or a beginner seeking an enjoyable recreational activity, pickleball offers an exhilarating experience filled with strategy, skill, and friendly competition. The combination of its unique court dimensions, paddle techniques, and lively gameplay makes pickleball an exceptional sport that continues to captivate players of all ages and skill levels worldwide.

Fast facts:

A "**pickler**" refers to an enthusiastic player or fan of pickleball. It is used to describe someone who enjoys and actively participates in the sport, showing a strong interest in and dedication to the game. Picklers are often passionate about pickleball and may be involved in playing, practicing, attending tournaments, or promoting the sport in various ways. The term "pickler" is a playful and informal way to describe individuals who have embraced the pickleball community and culture.

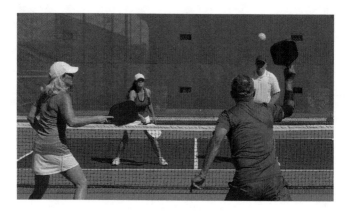

1.2   THE HISTORY OF PICKLEBALL

The history of pickleball can be traced back to the summer of 1965 when three friends—Joel Pritchard, Bill Bell, and Barney McCallum—created a unique game to keep their families entertained. Joel Pritchard, a U.S. Congressman from Washington State, and his friends found themselves in a bit of a predicament during a family gathering on Bainbridge Island.

As legend has it, Pritchard and his friend Bill Bell returned from a game of golf one day to find their kids bored and restless. With limited equipment available, they improvised by using a perforated plastic ball and lowered the badminton net to create a makeshift court. They used wooden paddles, similar to those used in table tennis, to volley the ball back and forth. This impromptu game became the foundation of what we now know as pickleball.

Fast facts:

The origins of the name "pickleball" have several theories. According to one popular account, Joel Pritchard's wife, Joan, named the game "pickleball" because it reminded her of the pickle boat in crew racing, where oarsmen were chosen from the leftovers of other boats. Another theory suggests that the name came from the Pritchards' dog, Pickles, who would often chase after the stray balls. Regardless of its origin, the name stuck, and pickleball was officially born.

After its humble beginnings, pickleball quickly gained popularity on Bainbridge Island. In the 1970s, pickleball began to spread beyond Washington State. Players introduced the game to neighboring regions, sparking interest, and attracting new enthusiasts. Tournaments and friendly matches were organized, creating opportunities for players to showcase their skills and compete against one another. The increased participation and enthusiasm for the sport further propelled its growth.

As more people discovered the game, they began modifying the rules and equipment to better suit their preferences. Originally, the game was played with ping pong paddles and a net that was only 36 inches high. Over time, the founders refined the rules and equipment used in the game, adapting it to be played on a regulation court with a lowered tennis net. Barney McCallum, one of the game's founders, made significant contributions to the sport by refining the rules and promoting its growth.

In 1972, the first pickleball tournament was held in Tukwila, Washington, with a small group of dedicated players. The sport continued to gain traction and drew the attention of enthusiasts beyond the Pacific Northwest.

The establishment of the **United States Pickleball Association (USAPA)** in 1984 marked a significant milestone in the evolution of pickleball. The USAPA became the governing body for the sport, setting official rules and regulations and promoting pickleball at the national level. With the formation of the USAPA, pickleball gained a structured framework that helped to standardize the game, ensuring consistency and fairness in competitions across the country.

Throughout the 1980s and 1990s, pickleball's popularity spread across the United States, particularly among older adults. The sport's low-impact nature, smaller court size, and slower pace made it appealing to individuals seeking a recreational activity that was easier on the joints but still offered an enjoyable workout.

Pickleball's international growth took off in the early 2000s, with the formation of the **International Federation of Pickleball (IFP)** in 2010. The IFP has since been instrumental in promoting pickleball worldwide, organizing international competitions, and supporting the sport's development in different countries. In recent years, pickleball has exploded in popularity, with players of all ages and skill levels embracing the fast-paced and engaging sport. It has become one of the fastest-growing sports, attracting players of all ages and skill levels.

According to a report by the Association of Pickleball Professionals, more than 36.5 million people played pickleball from August 2021 to August 2022. The sport is played in over 5,000 locations in the United States alone. It is also growing worldwide. The sport continues to evolve, with innovations in equipment, tournament formats, and the establishment of professional pickleball organizations.

Fast facts:

Did you know that **National Pickleball Day** is celebrated in the US on **August 8th** of each calendar year?

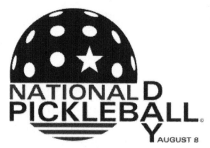

The idea of National Pickleball Day was dreamed up in 2021 by pickleball advocate, enthusiast and instructor, Deirdre Morris. This day celebrates and raises national awareness to the sport of pickleball and to encourage people to learn how to play the game.

Source: National Day Archives

In **Canada**, **National Pickleball Day** is celebrated on the **second Saturday of August** every year.

World Pickleball Day is celebrated annually on **October 10th**. The objective of World Pickleball Day is to establish pickleball as a game that is played across the world and not just North America. It is a day to promote the sport of pickleball to the general public by promoting the sport to new players and holding events to raise the profile of pickleball worldwide.

1.3   DISCOVERING THE BENEFITS OF PICKLEBALL

Let's dive into the top reasons why pickleball is capturing hearts and winning over players of all ages and backgrounds.

Top benefits of playing pickleball

✓ **Fun and engaging**: Pickleball is a fun and engaging sport that offers a unique combination of elements from different games. It's an incredibly enjoyable sport that offers a thrilling and engaging experience for players of all ages and skill levels. Whether you're a beginner or a seasoned athlete, the fast-paced rallies, strategic shots, and friendly competition will keep you entertained and coming back for more.

✓ **Quick learning curve**: Pickleball is easy to learn, with basic rules that can be picked up in a matter of minutes. This makes it an excellent introduction to racket sports for beginners. You'll be up and running in no time, enjoying the game, and improving your skills along the way. The simplicity of the game means you can quickly start playing and experience the joy of pickleball.

✓ **Suitable for all ages and skill levels**: Pickleball is a sport that can be played by anyone, regardless of age or skill level. It's an excellent way for families to bond over a shared activity, and it's also perfect for seniors looking for a low-impact sport to keep them active.

✓ **Family-friendly**: Bring the whole family together for a fun-filled activity. Pickleball is an excellent way to bond with loved ones of all generations. Whether you're playing with your kids, grandparents, or friends, everyone can join in the excitement and create cherished memories on the pickleball court.

✓ **Versatility**: Pickleball is a versatile sport that can be played in various settings. Whether you prefer indoor or outdoor play, there are plenty of options available. You can find dedicated pickleball courts, convert existing tennis courts, or set up a temporary court in your backyard. The flexibility of pickleball ensures you can enjoy the game wherever and whenever you want.

✓ **You can find many places to play**: One of the benefits of pickleball is the wide availability of places to play, with numerous dedicated courts and facilities found in communities, parks, and recreational centers. Whether you're a beginner or an experienced player, you can easily find convenient locations to enjoy the game and connect with fellow pickleball enthusiasts.

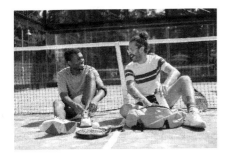
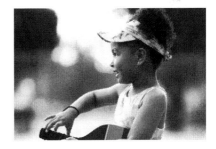

Pickleball is a popular sport that can be played in a variety of locations. The United States has over 15,000 pickleball courts and 5,000 venues where you can play pickleball. The country has only about 10,000 places to play, by USA Pickleball's count, but that continues to grow by several dozen every month. Dedicated pickleball courts are becoming more common, and many community centers, parks and recreation departments, and senior centers have courts available for use. In addition, tennis or badminton courts can easily be converted for pickleball play by adding temporary lines and adjusting the net height.

If you're looking for a place to play pickleball, you can start by checking with your local community center or parks and recreation department to see if they have courts available. You can also check with local sports clubs or organizations to see if they have pickleball facilities. In the USA, the **USA Pickleball Association** has a "Places to Play" feature on their website that allows you to search for pickleball courts near you.

In addition to dedicated courts and converted tennis or badminton courts, pickleball can also be played indoors in gymnasiums or other large spaces. Many schools and community centers have gymnasiums that can be used for pickleball play. Portable nets and temporary lines make it easy to set up a pickleball court in an indoor space.

✓ **Accessible year-round**: Pickleball can be played both indoors and outdoors, making it a sport that can be enjoyed year-round in any weather conditions. This makes it an excellent choice for anyone looking to stay active and healthy throughout the year.

✓ **The matches are often played quickly:** Pickleball matches are known for their fast-paced nature, with quick rallies and rapid exchanges adding excitement to the game. The combination of the court size, rules, and gameplay dynamics make pickleball matches highly engaging and ensure a thrilling experience for players.

How long do pickleball matches last? The length of a pickleball match can vary depending on the skill level of the players, the format of the match, and the number of games played. A typical game of pickleball usually lasts between 15 to 25 minutes. The game is played until one player or team reaches 11 points, with a margin of at least two points. However, some games may go longer if the teams are evenly matched or if there are many faults or rallies. In tournament play, matches are often the best two out of three games, which can take anywhere from 45 minutes to over an hour to complete.

✓ **Inexpensive**: Compared to other sports, pickleball is relatively inexpensive to play. The equipment required is minimal, and many parks and recreation centers offer free or affordable access to pickleball courts.

- ✓ **Social connection**: Pickleball is often played in doubles, which encourages teamwork and communication between players. Pickleball is a fantastic way to meet new people, build friendships, and be part of a vibrant community. Joining a pickleball club or participating in local events provides ample opportunities for social interaction and camaraderie. The bonds formed on the pickleball court often extend beyond the game, creating lifelong connections.
- ✓ **Fitness and health:** Pickleball is your ticket to elevating your fitness levels and enhancing your overall health. This dynamic sport offers a multitude of benefits, including a fantastic cardiovascular workout that gets your heart pumping. Not only does pickleball improve hand-eye coordination, but it also helps tone muscles, boost agility, and enhance both balance and flexibility. By engaging in regular pickleball sessions, you'll not only have a blast but also effectively maintain an active and healthy lifestyle. Plus, with the calories you'll burn and the opportunity to stay in shape, pickleball is the perfect choice for your physical well-being.
- ✓ **Low-impact, joint-friendly**: Don't let joint issues hold you back from staying active. Pickleball is a low-impact sport that minimizes stress on the joints, making it suitable for individuals of all ages and abilities. You can enjoy the benefits of exercise and competition without worrying about joint discomfort or injuries.
- ✓ **Mental stimulation**: Get ready to experience a mental workout like no other with pickleball. This exciting sport demands strategic thinking, quick decision-making, and the ability to anticipate your opponent's moves. By engaging in these mental challenges, you'll stimulate your brain, enhance cognitive function, and keep your mind sharp both on and off the court. Pickleball boosts mental agility through its requirement for quick thinking and strategic decision-making, leading to improved cognitive function, increased focus, and enhanced problem-solving skills. So, get your paddle ready and prepare to engage your mind in a thrilling game that not only tests your physical abilities but also keeps your mental acuity in top shape.
- ✓ **Stress relief**: Escape from the daily grind and let pickleball be your stress buster. The energetic gameplay and focus required on the court provide a welcome distraction and a chance to unwind. Playing pickleball releases endorphins, boosts your mood, and leaves you feeling refreshed and rejuvenated.
- ✓ **Lifelong learning and improvement**: Pickleball offers endless opportunities for personal growth and skill development. You'll constantly learn new techniques, refine your strategies, and discover ways to enhance your gameplay. The journey of improvement keeps you motivated, engaged, and always excited to take your pickleball skills to the next level.
- ✓ **Competitive opportunities:** For those looking to take their skills to the next level, pickleball offers numerous competitive opportunities, including local tournaments and professional leagues.

1.4   NAVIGATING THE COURT: LINES AND ZONES UNRAVELED

One of the first things you need to learn as a new pickleball player is the **dimensions and layout of the court**. This will help you position yourself effectively during the game, anticipate your opponent's shots, and move around the court efficiently. It's essential to understand the boundaries of the court to avoid stepping out of bounds during play. Understanding the court's layout will not only help you play the game correctly but also enhance your overall performance and enjoyment on the court.

Learning the court dimensions and layout is just the first step in becoming a proficient pickleball player. As you progress, you will discover various strategies and tactics that will enable you to make the most of the court's layout. So, take the time to study the court, practice your shots, and soon you'll be ready to take on opponents with confidence and skill.

Remember, pickleball is a game that can be enjoyed by players of all ages and skill levels. By understanding the court's dimensions and layout, you are well on your way to becoming a successful pickleball player. Get out there, have fun, and enjoy the exciting world of pickleball!

Understanding the dimensions and layout of the pickleball court

The **pickleball court** is a playing surface where the game of pickleball is played. The court has specific boundaries which dictate the playing area and determine the in-bounds and out-of-bounds shots.

Pickleball courts are rectangular in shape and measure 20 feet wide and 44 feet long.

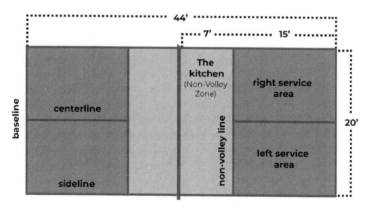

net height at sideline - 36 inches
(34 inches at center)

The court is divided into two equal halves by a 34-inch net, which is positioned at the center of the court's length. The net is slightly higher at the center, measuring 36 inches, and gradually slopes down to 34 inches at the posts.

Each half of the court is further divided into three sections: the **Non-Volley Zone (NVZ)**, the **mid-court area**, and the **baseline**.

Fast facts:

The pickleball court remains consistent for both singles and doubles play. However, in the variation known as **skinny singles**, players utilize only half the court with an imaginary line to close off the kitchen area. This modification creates narrower alleys on each side of the court, adding an extra level of difficulty as players must cover a reduced playing space and aim for precise shot placement. Other than this specific variation, the court dimensions, layout, and ball used are the same for both singles and doubles play. Skinny singles is an engaging game format that challenges players to adapt their strategies and showcase their skill in a more confined court, enhancing the excitement and competitiveness of the game.

Exploring the different lines and zones, such as the service court, baselines, sidelines, centerline and Non-Volley Zone (NVZ) and how they affect game play

Understanding the different lines and zones on the pickleball court is essential for players to navigate the playing area effectively and make strategic decisions during gameplay. Let's take a closer look at each of these elements and how they impact the game:

On either side of the net, there are two service courts and a 7-foot Non-Volley Zone or NVZ, (commonly referred to as "the kitchen,") extending from the net.

Service court:
Also known as the **service box**, the **service court** is the area on either side of the net where the ball must land when served. The service court is divided into two sections by the centerline, with each section measuring 10 feet wide by 15 feet long. The server must serve the ball diagonally, so that it lands in the service court diagonally opposite them. If the ball (serve) lands outside of the service court or in the Non-Volley Zone, it is considered a fault and results in a point for the receiving team.

Non-Volley Zone (the kitchen):
The **Non-Volley Zone** or **NVZ**, also known as the "**the kitchen**", is a seven-foot area on both sides of the net. It extends from the net to a line that is 15 feet away on each side. Players are not allowed to hit volleys (striking the ball before it bounces) while standing inside the Non-Volley Zone (NVZ). They can only enter this zone after the ball bounces, which adds an extra element of strategy to the game. This rule encourages strategic shot placement and prevents players from dominating the game with aggressive net play.

Mid-court area:
The **mid-court area** is located between the Non-Volley Zone (NVZ) and the baseline. This is where most of the rallies take place, and players have the opportunity to hit groundstrokes, lobs, and dinks. The baseline marks the end of the court, and players generally hit their serves and return shots from this area.

Baselines:
The **baselines** are the lines at the ends of the court, parallel to the net. They determine the depth of the court and play a significant role in serving and determining if a shot is in or out of play. Shots that land beyond the baselines are considered out.

Sidelines:
The **sidelines** run perpendicular to the net on each side of the court. They establish the width of the court and are essential for determining if a shot is in or out of bounds. Shots that land outside the sidelines are considered out.

Centerline:
The **centerline** is the line that divides the court into two equal halves. It serves as a reference point during gameplay, particularly for serving. The centerline also indicates the boundaries for each player's service area.

Understanding the layout and boundaries of the pickleball court is essential for players to position themselves effectively, make accurate line calls, and execute shots with precision. By staying within the boundaries and adhering to the rules associated with each area, players can maximize their gameplay and enjoy a fair and competitive game of pickleball.

Fast facts:

Nobody knows for certain why pickleball's **Non-Volley Zone** (**NVZ**) is called "**the kitchen**". However, there are a few popular theories. The term "kitchen" may have been borrowed from shuffleboard, where a similar term is used. In shuffleboard, the "kitchen" is an area behind the scoring zones where landing a shot results in a significant point deduction. As pickleball's creators drew inspiration from other leisure games, it's possible that they adopted the term from shuffleboard. Another theory suggests that the phrase "if you can't stand the heat, get out of the kitchen" may be relevant. With players from both teams positioned at the kitchen line, which is only 14 feet apart, the competition can become intense. Stepping into the kitchen to make a shot can add more pressure to the game, making rallies even more challenging and heated.

1.5   RULES AND SCORING: DECODING THE GAME

Pickleball is a dynamic sport with a set of rules that govern gameplay, ensuring fair and competitive matches. One of the aspects that makes pickleball such an exciting and accessible sport is its simple scoring system. Understanding the **basic rules** and **how to score** are crucial for players to engage in the game effectively. Here is an overview:

Overview of the basic rules of pickleball, including serving and scoring

The **USA Pickleball Association (USAPA)** and **International Federation of Pickleball (IFP)** publish the official rules for pickleball. Keep in mind that the rules of pickleball are subject to change and may vary depending on where you are playing. However, if you just want to get started, here are some of the basic rules that should apply in most cases:

In pickleball, the **starting server** is determined by a coin toss or rally. Really, any fair method will do. The winner of the coin toss or rally has the option to choose whether to serve first or to choose which side of the court to start on. Let's look at some of the basic rules:

Rule #1 Each pickleball game, and each point, begins with a serve

- A serve takes place behind the right service area, that is, behind the baseline and between the centerline and sideline. At the start of the game, the player on the right side (**even court**) serves to the receiving team by hitting the ball over the net to the diagonally opposite court. If a point is scored, the server moves to the left side (**odd court**) and serves to the diagonally opposite court.
- The serve must be made diagonally to the opposing service court, and the ball must clear the Non-Volley Zone (the kitchen), to be considered valid.
- If the ball lands on the sideline, baseline or centerline, the serve is considered in. If it lands on the Non-Volley line, it's a fault.

Note: Pickleball can be played as singles or doubles.

Starting player positions for pickleball doubles

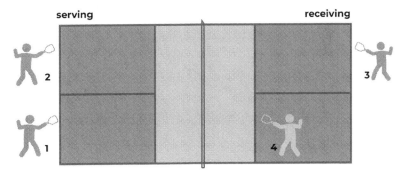

Serve placement – the serve must clear the NVZ (kitchen), including the line, to count

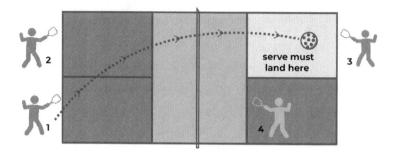

Rule #2 In pickleball, we have an underhand serve, or a drop serve, and that serve must go cross court.

- The server cannot touch the baseline or step into the court until the pickleball has been hit with the paddle using an **underhand serve** or **drop serve**, with the paddle striking the ball below the waist of the server. At the moment you strike the ball, neither foot can be inside the boundaries and at least one foot must be touching the ground behind the baseline. Both feet cannot be in the air.

Fast facts:

You can choose to hit the ball out of the air before it bounces or by dropping the ball with your non-paddle hand. In the case of the drop bounce, where you choose to hit it off a bounce, you cannot apply any upward or downward force to the ball. There is more detail about serving in **Chapter 4**.

You only get one chance to hit your serve in. If your serve lands in the NVZ (kitchen), the shot is hit out of bounds, or is hit into the net, you lose your serve and don't get to try again.

Fast facts:

With regard to serving, a **fault** occurs if:
- The serve does not clear the NVZ (kitchen), including the line.
- A shot is hit out of bounds, landing behind the baseline or outside the sideline.
- The shot is hit into the net. There is no "let" in pickleball. This means if the serve hits the net, there is no re-do (like in tennis).

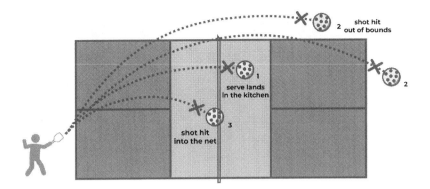

Rule #3 After the serve, each point continues until there is a fault

- The **receiver** allows the ball to bounce once before returning it.
- When the receiving team successfully returns the serve, the serving team must let the ball bounce once before hitting it.
- Once both teams have returned the ball successfully, the subsequent hits can be made either by volleying or allowing the ball to bounce once.
- A player can't return a ball that has been hit by the other team if it hasn't bounced in the Non-Volley Zone while standing in the Non-Volley Zone. The Non-Volley Zone restricts players from volleying the ball while standing within it.

Rule #4 You can hit groundstrokes in the kitchen, but you can't volley in the kitchen

The 7' zone on each side marks the Non-Volley Zone (NVZ) or kitchen.

- If your opponent hits a short shot that lands in the kitchen (a "**dink**"), you can enter and hit from the kitchen. However, it's important to note that once you have hit the ball while inside the kitchen, you must exit the kitchen without volleying the ball (hitting it out of the air) before your opponent's next shot.

As you will see in later chapters, a **dink** is a defensive shot and one of the most important parts of strategy in pickleball. One of the best moves after you've moved into the kitchen to field a dink is to dink right back to your opponent's kitchen.

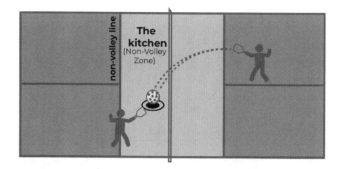

- You can never hit a **volley** (a short shot out of the air) while any part of your body is in the kitchen or even the kitchen line.
- In addition, you can't let your momentum carry you into the kitchen after you volley either.

There is a reason for this rule. Once a rally begins, players at the net have a huge advantage. They can hit any ball high enough with a downward 'smash'; this shot puts their opponents right on the defensive. Standing right on the net makes volleying too easy. So, the game's inventors took this unfair advantage away!

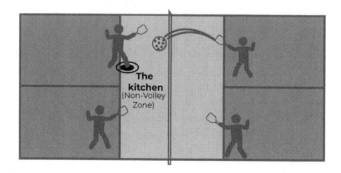

Rule #5 The ball must bounce on both sides before either team can volley

- Before any player can **volley** (hit a shot out of the air), the ball must bounce at least once on each side.

If your partner is serving and you start up at the kitchen, you are in a dangerous position. This is because your opponents can hit a ball straight at you and, if you react with a volley, that's a fault and you lose a point.

This rule keeps the serving team back at the baseline to start. Without this rule, the serving team could easily rush the net, giving them an unfair edge every time. The returning team would struggle to ever regain the serve and get points.

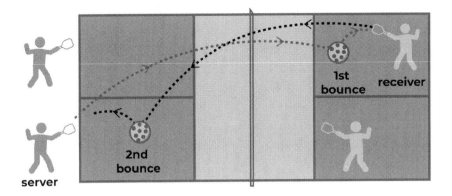

Rule #6 Only the serving team can score points

- In pickleball, you only win points on your serve, and you continue serving until you lose a point.
- Games are typically played to 11 or 15 points, and the serving team continues to serve until they lose a **rally**.
- A point is earned when the receiving team fails to return the ball or commits a fault.
- After winning each point on your serve, you switch sides with your partner and serve to the other opponent.
- The serving team serves until it faults, alternating between right and left service areas. This means, if you win the rally as the serving team, you win the point, switch side of the court and the same server will serve, but in the opposite direction. The receiving team does not alternate positions.
- If you lose the rally as the serving team, then the serve moves to the next player. If the serve goes to the other side of the court (called a **side out**), then, in doubles play, the person on the right-hand side of the court will go first. In singles pickleball you will serve on the side of the court based on your score.
- If the receiving team wins a rally, they gain the serve, but no points are awarded. The serving team continues to accumulate points until they fault, allowing the opposing team to take over the serve and have an opportunity to score.
- The serving team's point score will always be an even number when the serving team's starting server is serving on the right hand side of the court. A team's score will always be an odd number when their team's starting server is serving from the left-hand side of the court.

In **doubles pickleball**, the first serving team only has one service turn. So, if the serving team loses the first rally, then the serve goes to the other team. After this first side out, each side has two service turns. In other words, each player gets a shot at serving.

In pickleball, the score is called out before each serve:

- In **doubles play**, the score is made up of three numbers, with the first number representing the serving team's score, the second number representing the receiving team's score, and the third number representing the server number (either 1 or 2). For example, a score of 3-2-1 means that the serving team has 3 points, the receiving team has 2 points, and it is server #1's turn to serve.
- In **singles play**, the score is made up of only two numbers, with the first number representing the server's score and the second number representing the receiver's score. For example, a score of 3-2 means that the server has 3 points and the receiver has 2 points.

Explanation of fault, let, and side out

Fault:
- A fault occurs when a player fails to comply with the rules, resulting in a loss of the rally and a point for the opposing team.
- Common faults include stepping into the Non-Volley Zone (the kitchen) while volleying, volleying the ball before it bounces, hitting the ball out of bounds, and serving into the wrong service court.

Let:
- A let occurs when there is interference or an unintended hindrance during play, such as a ball hitting the net and still landing in the correct service area.
- In the case of a let, the point is replayed without penalty.

Side out:
- A side out occurs when the serving team loses a rally, and the receiving team gains the serve.
- This usually happens when the serving team commits a fault, hits the ball out of bounds, or fails to return the ball.

Understanding the double bounce rule and Non-Volley Zone violation

Double bounce rule:
- The double bounce rule is a fundamental rule in pickleball that ensures fair play and equal opportunities for both teams.
- According to this rule, each team must let the ball bounce once on each side before volleys (hitting the ball in the air) are allowed.
- The serving team starts the point with an underhand serve, and the receiving team must let the serve bounce before returning it.
- After the serve, both teams must let the ball bounce once on each side before volleys are permitted.
- Once the ball has bounced on both sides, players have the option to volley or play the ball off a bounce.
- The double bounce rule encourages longer rallies, strategic shot placement, and prevents overly aggressive net play.

Non-Volley Zone violation:
- The Non-Volley Zone, also known as the kitchen, is a designated area near the net where players are not allowed to volley the ball.
- The Non-Volley Zone extends seven feet on each side of the net and is marked by a line.
- Players must keep both feet behind the Non-Volley Zone line when volleying the ball.
- Violating the Non-Volley Zone by stepping into it or hitting a volley from within it results in a fault, and the opposing team gains the serve.
- The Non-Volley Zone violation rule promotes fair play, encourages strategic shot selection, and prevents players from dominating the game with constant net play.

Understanding and adhering to the double bounce rule and Non-Volley Zone violation is crucial for players to maintain a fair and competitive game. By following these rules, players can showcase their skills, engage in exciting rallies, and enjoy the dynamic nature of pickleball. It is important to practice these rules during gameplay, seek clarification when needed, and respect the integrity of the game.

Introduction to the concept of side changes and alternating serves

Side changes:
- In pickleball, side changes occur at the end of each game and during **tiebreak** situations.
- After completing a game, players switch sides of the court to ensure fairness and equal playing conditions.
- Side changes also occur when the total number of points played reaches an odd number, typically 7 or 11, during a game.
- Switching sides allows players to experience and adapt to different court conditions, such as sun direction, wind, and surface variations.
- Side changes promote fairness and help negate any potential advantage or disadvantage associated with specific court conditions.

Alternating serves:

In pickleball doubles, each team has two servers. The **first server** serves until their team loses a rally. Then, the serve passes to the second server on the team (the **second server**). The second server continues to serve until their team commits a fault and loses the serve to the other team. The second server is the partner of the first server and will serve from their correct side of the court if the first server loses a serve.

- In pickleball, the serving team must alternate their serves between players on the serving team.
- The first serve of each game starts from the right-hand service court, and subsequent serves switch between the left and right service courts.
- When the serving team wins a rally, they earn a point. When you win a point, you and your partner swap sides of the court (right and left). You never serve in the same direction, or to the same opponent, twice in a row.

- When the serving team makes a fault and loses the rally, the first server is no longer allowed to continue serving. Instead, their partner becomes the second server and gets the chance to serve. There is an exception: if the serving team wins the first rally, the first server remains the server until they lose a rally. Since the serving team did not win a point, the partners do not switch positions and remain in their current locations.
- The second server continues serving, alternating sides, until their team loses another rally. That team now has run out of chances to serve.
- It is now the other team's turn to serve and try and win some points.
- After the serving team loses a rally and the opposing team gains the serve, the new serving team must start from the right-hand service court.
- When a **side out** occurs, the player who is standing on the right side of the court for the new serving team begins serving. They continue serving and winning points until their team commits a fault and loses the rally.
- Then their partner starts serving, from whatever side they happen to be standing on, until their team commits a second fault, resulting in a side out back to the other team.

Alternating serves ensure that each player on the serving team has an equal opportunity to contribute to the game and prevents any player from dominating the serving duties.

It is also a rule that before you can serve, you must announce the score or call out all three numbers of the score. This is known as "**calling the score**". Call your own team's score first, your opponents' score second, and then either a "one" or a "two", depending on whether you are the first or second serve for that round.

Basic pickleball line call rules

Shots on the lines of the pickleball court are "**in**", with one exception – the Non-Volley Zone line on the serve is "**out**".

The basic pickleball **line call rules** are:

- The pickleball must land in the correct service court on the serve. All of the lines of the correct service court, except for the Non-Volley Zone line (kitchen line) are "**in**". So, if the service pickleball lands on the sideline, centerline or baseline, the serve is "**in**". If the pickleball serve lands in the Non-Volley Zone, on the Non-Volley Zone line, or completely outside of the lines of the service court, then the serve is "**out**".
- On any shot, other than the serve, the pickleball in "**in**" if it lands anywhere on the pickleball court. This includes all of the lines of the pickleball court. So, if the pickleball lands on the sideline, centerline, baseline, or the Non-Volley Zone line on any shot, other than the serve, then the pickleball is "**in**." If the pickleball lands completely outside of the lines on the pickleball court, then the pickleball is "**out**."
- If the pickleball is "**in**", the rally continues on. If the pickleball is "**out**", then the player (singles) or team (doubles) that hit the pickleball out of bounds would have committed a fault and loses the rally.

- "**Out**" calls are made by the pickleball players on the side of the pickleball court where the pickleball bounces.

Examples of scoring in doubles:

In each turn, both players get the opportunity to serve. In pickleball (doubles) scoring, you will hear players announce three numbers – "**Zero, zero...two**". That third number tracks which of the two players on a team has the serve.

For example, let's say that the game is tied at **5-5**. If you start the serve (from the right-hand side), you'll announce, "**5-5-1**". This is so everyone knows that you are the first player in rotation serving.

Then, let's say you lose the point, the ball doesn't go to your opponents. It goes to your teammate who will announce "**5-5-2**".

If your partner loses their serve, the ball goes back to your opponents, who will announce "**5-5-1**". Your team will need to win points on both opponents' serves to get the ball back. The game continues until one team gets **11 points**. However, you have to win by **2**.

Let's imagine that the game is tied **10-10**. The next score doesn't win. The game continues past **11-10**. You can have ending scores of **12-10**, **15-13**, or **21-19**, for example.

This rule means that games can go on for a long time, but it also adds to the fun and excitement!

Fast facts:

An exception to the rules! Remember that at the beginning of game, the first team to serve was chosen at random (such as a coin toss). That team only gets one chance to serve for that round, rather than the usual two. This prevents them from racking up lots of points before the other team has the opportunity to serve and score. For that reason, the opening score of pickleball game is actually **0-0-2** not **0-0-1**. As soon as the original serving team commits a fault, it's a side out, and the other team gets to serve. From this point on, both teams get two chances to serve on every round.

Singles rules and scoring

In singles pickleball, the game is played between two players on opposite sides of the court. As with doubles, the objective of the game is to score points by hitting the ball over the net and into the opponent's court without them being able to return it.

The serving and scoring rules are slightly different from doubles.

How do you know what side of the court to serve in pickleball singles? In singles, the serve is always taken from the **right side** of the court when the server has an **even number** (0, 2, 4, 6, 8 or 10 points) and from the **left side** when the server has an **odd number** (1, 3, 5, 7 or 9 points).

Serving positions in pickleball singles

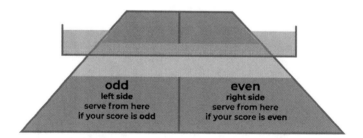

Serving:

- The **first server** is determined by a coin toss or other agreed-upon method.
- The server stands behind the baseline and serves diagonally to the opponent's service court.

- The serve must clear the Non-Volley Zone (kitchen) and land in the diagonally opposite service court.
- If the serve is successful, the server's score starts at "0" and they continue serving.

Scoring:

- Scoring in singles pickleball follows the **traditional** or **side-out scoring system** is used. This means that points can only be scored by the serving player. The receiving player cannot score points.
- A point is scored by serving the ball and winning the rally, meaning that the opponent is unable to return the ball or hits it out of bounds.
- If the server wins the rally, they score a point and continue to serve.
- The server continues to serve until they make a fault, such as hitting the ball out of bounds or into the net. When this happens, the serve passes to the other player, who then becomes the server. If the serve is a fault, it results in a side out, and the opponent becomes the server.
- The new server then serves the ball and the sequence repeats.
- Games are typically played to 11 points, and a two-point advantage is required to win. In case of a 10-10 tie, the game continues until one player has a two-point lead.

In **summary** for **singles**:

1. The first serve for each side starts on the right-hand side.
2. If the server wins the point, the server switches sides of the court.
3. If the receiver wins the point, neither player switches sides.
4. The server continues until they lose a point.
5. There is only one serve per rotation. If the server loses a point, the serve goes to the receiver.

There is no second server. So, if you lose the point on your serve, it goes straight to your opponent.

It is only the server's score that determines which side to serve from and not the combined score of the server and receiver.

Differences between singles and doubles:

With a few exceptions. singles pickleball generally has the same rules as doubles pickleball. For instance, the pickleball rules for serving, the Non-Volley Zone, line calls, and faults all apply to singles pickleball in the same manner as doubles pickleball.

The main differences between singles and doubles in pickleball lie in the number of players on each side and the serving and receiving positions. In doubles, there are two players on each side, forming a team, and both players have the opportunity to serve before a side out occurs. In singles, there is only one player on each side, and the serving player serves until a fault is made. The serving and receiving positions are distinct in singles as compared to doubles.

In doubles, players often adopt specific roles as either the server or the receiver, alternating their positions after each point. They work together as a team to cover the court and strategically position themselves to capitalize on their opponents' weaknesses. Communication and coordination between teammates are crucial in doubles play.

On the other hand, singles players are responsible for covering the entire court individually. They must possess strong footwork, agility, and the ability to cover the court efficiently. Strategies in singles revolve around creating and exploiting openings, employing various shot placements, and using court coverage to their advantage.

Overall, the dynamics of the game, court coverage, and strategies differ between singles and doubles in pickleball. Understanding these differences can help players adjust their playing style, positioning, and tactics to excel in either format.

Fast facts:

In pickleball, the **tiebreak** is a method used to determine the winner of a set that has reached a tied score. It is typically employed when the score reaches a certain threshold, such as 10-10 or 15-15, depending on the agreed-upon rules. During a tiebreak, each team or player takes turns serving for one point at a time. The team or player who reaches a predetermined number of points, usually 7 or 11, and leads by at least two points, wins the tiebreak and the set. The tiebreak is an exciting and decisive phase of the game, adding intensity and suspense to the match while providing a fair way to determine the winner of a closely contested set.

The rally scoring system

There has been some discussion in the pickleball community about the possibility of changing the scoring system to rally scoring. **Rally scoring** is a scoring system used in some sports where a point is awarded on every rally, regardless of which team is serving. This means that a point is scored on every play, and the game can move more quickly.

There are pros and cons to using rally scoring. One advantage is that it can make games faster and more exciting, as points are scored more frequently. It can also reduce the impact of a strong server, as points can be scored by either team regardless of who is serving. The traditional scoring system allows for more strategy and control over the game.

However, the current official rules of pickleball, as set by organizations such as the USA Pickleball Association and the International Federation of Pickleball, specify that the **traditional** or **side-out scoring system** must be used. This means that points can only be scored by the serving team, and the receiving team cannot score points. The server continues to serve until they make a fault, at which point the serve passes to the other player. A point is scored by serving the ball and winning the rally. This is the official scoring system used in all sanctioned pickleball games and tournaments.

1.6 PICKLEBALL SKILL RATING

What is meant by pickleball skill rating? A **pickleball skill rating** is a system used to assess and categorize players based on their skill level in the game. It provides a standardized way to measure and communicate a player's proficiency and helps ensure fair competition among players of similar abilities.

The skill rating is typically represented by a number or a combination of letters and numbers, such as 2.5, 3.0, 3.5, etc. The rating scale usually ranges from beginner-level (lower numbers) to advanced-level (higher numbers).

The rating is determined through various factors, including technical skills, strategy, shot selection, consistency, court positioning, and overall game performance. It considers both offensive and defensive abilities, as well as the player's understanding of the rules and their ability to adapt to different game situations.

Skill ratings are often used in tournaments, leagues, and organized play to ensure balanced and competitive matchups. By assigning players to appropriate skill levels, it promotes enjoyable and fair gameplay where players can compete against opponents of similar abilities.

For **beginners**, skill ratings provide a benchmark to assess their progress and help set goals for improvement. As you gain experience and enhance your skills, your rating can increase over time. It's important to remember that skill ratings are not definitive labels but rather a tool to guide players and facilitate fair competition.

It is common for beginners to start with lower skill ratings and gradually progress as they develop their techniques, gain experience, and become more confident in their gameplay. Don't be discouraged by your initial rating but instead see it as an opportunity to learn, grow, and work towards advancing your skills in the exciting sport of pickleball.

Different pickleball skill rating systems

So, how do you know what your pickleball skill rating is or how to improve that rating? According to **pickleheads.com**, your pickleball rating is a gauge of how good you are at the game and there are several different ways that your ability can be assessed and ranked.

The pickleball "**self-rating**" system. In this method, you give yourself a skill rating between 1.0 and 6.0, based on certain criteria. Check out – pickleheads.com/guides/pickleball-rating

The **USA Pickleball** association (**USAPA**) publishes a list of guidelines on how you should score yourself. The score you get depends on the skills you have mastered. The pickleball ratings chart and a simplified chart are in the **APPENDIX – QUICK REFERENCE GUIDE**.

General pickleball skill levels. According to **pickleheads.com**, if you're not ready yet to give yourself a score out of 6, there is a simpler system known as the "**general pickleball skill level**". Here, you are given three options:

- **Beginners**: These range from those who are playing for the first time to players who can sustain a short rally and are starting to try out some backhand shots. These players would range from **1.0 to 3.5**. They can hit simple shots and have a basic understanding of the rules and strategy.
- **Intermediate**: These are players with a rating of around **4.0 to 4.5**. They understand the rules and strategy and can sustain a rally using a combination of shots, including backhands. Intermediate players can hit shots with good spin and don't make too many unforced errors. This group is probably the largest at your local club or league.
- **Advanced**: Mastered the game. Use advanced strategies. Experienced in competitive play. Rating level **5.0 and above**.

Intermediate players are more likely to be intimidated by the idea of playing against them. They are able to spot weaknesses in their opponents and target them with precision. Advanced players can execute all types of shots consistently and they understand the finer tactics of the game.

Many clubs and leagues use these classifications because it is a great way to divide up the players who will enjoy playing together and have fun.

Fast facts:

The **USA Pickleball Player Skill Ratings rubric** provides specific skills that need to be achieve each level of player ratings. If you go to the URL below, you can either click on any of the toggles to display a specific definition of each rating level or download a PDF version.

usapickleball.org/tournaments/tournament-player-ratings/player-skill-rating-definitions/

Top tips:

How can you improve your pickleball skills rating?

- ✓ Do practice drills
- ✓ Watch tutorial videos
- ✓ Take lessons
- ✓ Play against higher-rated players
- ✓ Improve your game

USA Pickleball Tournament Player Ratings (**UTPR**), formerly known as "USAPA pickleball ratings" is a rating system based solely on a player's previous performances in pickleball tournaments, that is, playing history. Only members of USA Pickleball that compete in competitions can have a UTPR. UTPR scores range from 0.000 to 6.999. Essentially, when you win, your score goes up and down when you lose. However, a player's score only changes when they play sanctioned, official tournaments.

Fast facts:

USA Pickleball, the official governing body in pickleball in the U.S. and the leading pickleball tournament software company, **pickleballtournaments.com**, have created a **player rating system** to help tournament directors and players improve their tournament experience.

Go to **USA Pickleball** for more information – usapickleball.org/tournaments/tournament-player-ratings/

Finally, there is the "**Dreamland (Dynamic) Universal Pickleball Ratings**". This system was devised by Steve Kuhn, the owner of Dreamland, a pickleball entertainment centre near Austin, Texas.

Also known as the **DUPR**, as it is known, is a new pickleball rating system that embraces a freer way of calculating a player's ranking. In this system, a player can self-report their own wins and losses in any matches they play providing one other player verifies the result. So, every match a player plays is counted towards their pickleball rating, even though they might never play an official tournament. All someone needs to do is report their wins and losses to DUPR and their rating will be calculated. A **DUPR rating** ranges from 2.000 to 8.000 and is based on the same **Elo rating system** as the UTPR.

What is the **DUPR** and how does it work? According to **mydupr.com**, Dynamic Universal Pickleball Rating is the most accurate and only global rating system in Pickleball. All players, regardless of their age, gender, location, or skill, are rated on the same scale between 2.0-8.0 based on their match results.

DUPR is free and anyone can have a rating. One match result is all it takes to have a DUPR rating, and 5-10 match results is all it takes to have an even more accurate rating. If you've ever played in a Pickleball tournament you most likely already have a DUPR rating and can claim your account at mydupr.com or by downloading the iOS or Android app.

DUPR is a modified **Elo algorithm** that uses a player's last rating to update their new rating. The algorithm considers three factors:

1. **Victory**: Did you win or lose? If you win your rating will go up and if you lose, your rating will go down.
2. **Type of Result**: Was this a self-posted rec play score, a league match, or a sanctioned tournament result? Rec play will count less towards your rating change.
3. **Rating Difference of Opponent**: If your opponent is rated higher than you and you win, you'll increase more than if your opponent is lower rated and vice versa.

Go to mydupr.com for more details.

What is the **Elo rating system**? The Elo rating system is a widely used method in competitive games, including pickleball, to assess and compare players' skill levels. In the context of pickleball, the Elo system assigns a numerical rating to each player, representing their relative proficiency in the sport. When two players with different Elo ratings compete against each other, the outcome of the match will lead to an adjustment of their respective ratings.

If a lower-rated player defeats a higher-rated player in a pickleball match, the lower-rated player will gain more Elo points than if they defeated a player of similar rating. Conversely, if a higher-rated player defeats a lower-rated player, they will only gain a few points. This mechanism helps maintain the accuracy of the rating system and allows it to reflect the actual skill levels of players over time.

The Elo rating system is particularly useful in tournaments, as it helps in seeding players. Higher-rated players are typically placed in higher brackets, while lower-rated players are positioned in lower brackets, ensuring more balanced and competitive matches throughout the tournament. The system also facilitates fair and challenging matches during casual play, as players of similar skill levels are more likely to compete against each other.

There are several organizations that rank pickleball players.

- **USA Pickleball (USAP)**, which uses the UTPR (USA Pickleball Tournament Player Ratings) system.
- **The Professional Pickleball Association (PPA)**, which prefers the DUPR (Dreamland Universal Pickleball Rating) system.
- **Association of Pickleball Professionals (APP)**, the Pro Tour Partner of USAP, who also prefers the DUPR system for ranking players.
- **World Pickleball Rankings (WPR)**, which has worked with all of the major pickleball organizations to try and consolidate ranks.
- **Global Pickleball Rankings (GPR)**, managed by Pickleball Global, are rankings that are age-based and a player's best 15 event results over the past year.

Check out the **APPENDIX – PICKLEBALL RATINGS AND RANKINGS** for more information.

1.7   READ, WATCH AND LEARN: OBSERVING PICKLEBALL IN ACTION

While reading about the fundamentals of pickleball is essential, witnessing the game in action can greatly enhance your understanding and learning experience. Observing pickleball being played allows you to see the concepts and techniques in practice, providing valuable insights and inspiration for your own gameplay. There are several ways to see pickleball in action.

Top tips:

As you read through this book, find a **video** (there are lots of great resources to get you started in the section – **RESOURCES FOR IMPROVING YOUR GAME**) that corresponds to what you are learning about. In other word, **READ WATCH LEARN**!

Here are a few ways you can watch pickleball in action and enrich your learning journey:

- **Attend local pickleball events**: Look for local pickleball tournaments, leagues, or casual play sessions in your area. Watching live games will give you a firsthand experience of the sport, allowing you to observe different playing styles, strategies, and the dynamics of the game. You can also interact with experienced players, ask questions, and learn from their expertise.
- **Join pickleball clubs**: Joining a local pickleball club or community is an excellent way to immerse yourself in the game. These clubs often organize regular playing sessions, where you can watch and participate in matches. Being a part of a pickleball community provides opportunities to observe skilled players, receive guidance, and engage in friendly competition.

- **Online videos and tutorials**: The internet offers a vast array of pickleball videos, tutorials, and match highlights. Platforms like YouTube and social media platforms are treasure troves of pickleball content. Watch instructional videos from renowned players and coaches, as well as exciting match footage. By observing the techniques, strategies, and shot selection of experienced players, you can gain valuable insights to incorporate into your own game.
- **Live streaming and broadcasts**: Stay updated with live streaming events and televised pickleball matches. Some professional pickleball tournaments and major events are broadcast online or on sports channels. Watching high-level competitive matches will expose you to advanced strategies, intense rallies, and the skills of top players. Take note of their positioning, shot variety, and decision-making under pressure.

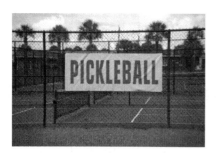 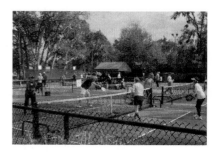

Should I get a coach?

As a new pickleball player, getting a coach can be a great way to improve your skills and progress in the game. A coach can help to correct mechanics or strategic problems, customize their lessons according to your needs, and provide strategic advice and practice skills that they recommend.

When searching for a coach, it is advisable to check if they hold certification from recognized organizations, as it ensures they have undergone training and demonstrated their expertise in teaching pickleball. Pickleball coaches can become certified through various organizations that offer training and certification programs. For example, in the US, the **USA Pickleball Association (USAPA)** offers a certification program for instructors. To become certified, coaches must pass two continuing education units per year and meet other requirements. Other organizations, such as the **International Pickleball Teaching Professional Association (IPTPA)** and the **Professional Pickleball Registry (PPR)**, also offer certification programs for pickleball coaches.

However, certification should not be the sole factor in selecting a coach. Equally important is finding someone with experience instructing players at your skill level, effective communication skills, and a teaching style that aligns with your learning style.

To find a suitable coach, consider seeking recommendations from other players or consulting local pickleball clubs and organizations for a list of certified coaches. Look for coaches who possess in-depth knowledge of the game and can effectively communicate with you based on your learning preferences.

To locate a coach, you can initiate an online search for pickleball coaches in your area. Additionally, reach out to local sports clubs, community centers, or parks and recreation departments to inquire about pickleball lessons or recommended coaches. Some coaches may also offer group lessons or clinics, which can be a more cost-effective option compared to private lessons.

Top tips:

Clinics or private lesson? What is recommended for beginners?

For **beginners in pickleball**, both clinics and private lessons have their benefits. Here are some considerations to help you decide:

Clinics:
Clinics are group sessions led by experienced instructors, where multiple players can learn and practice together. They provide an opportunity to learn from others, observe different playing styles, and engage in drills and game scenarios. Clinics are often structured with specific focuses, such as fundamentals, strategies, or specific shots, allowing beginners to gain a comprehensive understanding of the game. Clinics can be more affordable than private lessons and offer a social and supportive environment for learning and interacting with other players.

Private lessons:
Private lessons involve one-on-one instruction with a coach or instructor. They offer personalized attention and tailored guidance to address specific areas of improvement for the individual player. Private lessons can be beneficial for beginners who prefer a more individualized approach, allowing them to receive immediate feedback, focused skill development, and personalized training plans. Private lessons can also be flexible in terms of scheduling and can progress at the player's own pace.

The choice between clinics and private lessons ultimately depends on your preferences, learning style, and budget. If you enjoy learning in a group setting, want to interact with other players, and have a more budget-friendly option, clinics can be a great choice. On the other hand, if you prefer individualized attention, personalized feedback, and focused skill development, private lessons may be the better option for you. Some beginners may even choose to combine both approaches, taking part in clinics to learn the basics and then supplementing with private lessons to refine specific skills.

Regardless of your choice, seeking guidance from experienced instructors or coaches can greatly accelerate your learning curve and help you build a strong foundation in pickleball.

Once you have chosen a coach, it is crucial to clearly communicate your goals and aspirations for coaching. This allows your coach to tailor their lessons to your specific needs, facilitating your progress in the game. Consistent practice is equally important, as it enables you to apply the skills and techniques learned during lessons.

Overall, investing in a coach can greatly enhance your development as a pickleball player. Working with an experienced and knowledgeable coach empowers you to improve your skills, acquire new techniques, and advance in the game.

CHAPTER 2   GEAR ESSENTIALS

One of the great things about pickleball is that it doesn't require a lot of fancy equipment or gear to get started. As a new pickleball player, you'll only need a few essential items to begin enjoying the game.

In **Chapter 2**, we will delve into the fundamental components that play a crucial role in enhancing your pickleball experience. From finding the perfect paddle to selecting the right ball, dressing for optimal performance, and choosing the ideal footwear, we will explore the gear essentials that will elevate your game to new heights.

2.1   PADDLE POWER: FINDING YOUR PERFECT MATCH

In the world of pickleball, the **paddle** is your ultimate companion on the court. Just as a tennis player relies on a racket, a pickleball player depends on their paddle to make precise shots and engage in thrilling rallies. The paddle is similar to a large table tennis paddle and is used to hit the ball over the net.

The pickleball paddle is a specially designed instrument crafted from a variety of materials such as wood, composite, or graphite, each offering different levels of control and power. The paddle features a handle for grip, a paddle face for striking the ball, and a core that determines the paddle's weight and responsiveness. The paddle's unique construction and characteristics greatly influence your gameplay, allowing you to control the ball's trajectory, generate power, and execute precise shots.

Types of pickleball paddles and their characteristics (weight, grip size, material)

When it comes to pickleball, choosing the right paddle is essential for beginners. A well-suited paddle can greatly enhance your gameplay and overall enjoyment of the sport.

Understanding the weight, grip size, and materials of a pickleball paddle is crucial as it allows players to find a paddle that complements their playing style, provides optimal control and power, and ultimately enhances their overall performance on the court.

Weight:
Pickleball paddles come in various weights, ranging from lightweight to heavyweight.
- Lightweight paddles (around 6-7 ounces) offer increased maneuverability and quick swings, suitable for players seeking speed and control.
- Midweight paddles (around 7-8.5 ounces) strike a balance between power and control, appealing to a wide range of players.
- Heavyweight paddles (above 8.5 ounces) provide more power and stability, making them suitable for players who prefer a stronger and more aggressive game.

For a beginner, it is recommended to start with a lighter paddle, typically between 6.5 to 8 ounces. A lighter paddle allows for easier maneuverability and control, helping you develop your strokes and techniques effectively.

Grip size:
Pickleball paddles have different grip sizes to accommodate players' hand sizes and personal preferences.
- Smaller grip sizes (4 inches) offer more control and maneuverability, ideal for players with smaller hands or those who prefer a tighter grip.
- Standard grip sizes (4.25 inches) are the most common and suitable for a wide range of players.
- Larger grip sizes (4.5 inches) provide added comfort and support for players with larger hands or those who prefer a looser grip.

It should fit comfortably in your hand, allowing for a secure grasp and minimizing the risk of injury. Beginners often find a grip size of 4.25 inches to be suitable, but it ultimately depends on your hand size and personal preference.

Material:
Pickleball paddles are made from different materials, each offering unique characteristics.
- **Composite** paddles, made from layered materials such as fiberglass or carbon fiber, provide a blend of power, control, and durability. They offer a good balance between durability and performance.
- **Wood** paddles, typically made from hardwood or composite wood, offer excellent touch, feel, and control. Wooden paddles are the most affordable option but tend to be heavier and less durable.
- **Graphite** paddles are known for their lightweight nature, providing excellent control and power.

For a beginner, a composite paddle is a popular choice due to its versatility and affordability.

Fast facts:

Paddles come in different **shapes**, such as oval, elongated, and traditional. The shape you choose depends on your playstyle and comfort. Traditional-shaped paddles are commonly recommended for beginners as they provide a larger sweet spot and more forgiveness on off-center hits.

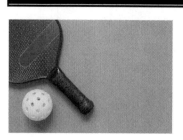
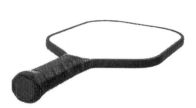

According to **pickleballcentral.com**, manufacturers design pickleball paddles utilizing a variety of materials and technologies intended to add the elements of either **power** or **control**. It is the combination of all the factors – shape, core, face, handle and weight – which translate to specific play characteristics on the court.

- **Power paddles** tend to have hotter and tighter sweet spots and provide greater feedback. Power elements: elongated shape, thinner core, fiberglass face, longer handle, heavier weights.
- **Control paddles** tend to have larger and more consistent sweet spots and are forgiving of mis-hits. Control elements: wider or rounder shape, thicker core, graphite or carbon fiber face, traditional length or shorter handle, lighter weights.

The circumference of the grip is more about comfort than power or control. You want to find a grip that works best for your hand size.

What is an edgeless paddle? An **edgeless paddle** in pickleball is a paddle that does not have an edge guard around the perimeter of the paddle face. The edge guard is a protective strip that is typically made of plastic or rubber and is designed to protect the paddle from damage when it comes into contact with the ground or other hard surfaces. Edgeless paddles, on the other hand, do not have this protective strip and instead have a smooth, uninterrupted playing surface that extends all the way to the edge of the paddle. This design allows for a larger sweet spot and more responsive play, as there is no interruption in the playing surface. However, edgeless paddles may be more prone to damage if they come into contact with hard surfaces.

Price is an important consideration for beginners. While it may be tempting to opt for the cheapest paddle available, investing in a mid-range paddle can greatly enhance your experience. Quality paddles within the $50 to $100 range offer better control, durability, and overall performance compared to entry-level options.

Choosing the right paddle based on playing style and skill level

When it comes to choosing the right paddle for your pickleball game, there are several factors to consider. Whether you're a beginner or an experienced player, finding a paddle that suits your playing style and preferences can make a significant difference in your performance on the court.

Tips for new players:

✓ **Determine your playing style**: Consider whether you prefer control or power-based shots and choose a paddle that aligns with your style.
✓ **Try different paddle weights**: Experiment with paddles of varying weights to find one that feels comfortable and easy to maneuver.
✓ **Consider grip size**: Select a paddle with a grip size that allows you to hold it securely and comfortably during gameplay.
✓ **Evaluate paddle materials**: Choose a paddle made of durable materials like graphite or composite for longevity and performance.
✓ **Seek advice from experienced players**: Consult with more experienced pickleball players or coaches to get recommendations on paddle selection.
✓ **Read product reviews**: Look for reviews and testimonials from other players to gain insights into the performance and quality of different paddles.
✓ **Demo paddles**: Take advantage of paddle demo programs offered by pickleball clubs or stores to try out different paddles before making a purchase.
✓ **Set a budget**: Determine your budget range and find a paddle that offers a good balance of quality and affordability.
✓ **Prioritize comfort**: Choose a paddle that feels comfortable in your hand and allows for easy control of shots.
✓ **Take your time**: Don't rush your decision. Take the time to research and try out different paddles to find the one that suits your needs and playing style best.

Tips for more experienced players:

✓ **Assess your playing style**: Analyze your strengths and weaknesses to identify the specific paddle characteristics that will enhance your game.
✓ **Consider paddle shape**: Explore different paddle shapes, such as traditional or elongated, and understand how they can affect shot control and reach.
✓ **Evaluate core materials**: Look into paddle cores made of materials like polymer or aluminum honeycomb, which can impact power and control.
✓ **Experiment with surface textures**: Try paddles with different surface textures, such as smooth or textured, to find the one that provides optimal ball spin and control.
✓ **Fine-tune weight distribution:** Customize the weight distribution of your paddle by adding or removing grip wraps or modifying the handle for better balance.
✓ **Keep an eye on paddle technology**: Stay updated on the latest paddle technologies and innovations that can improve your performance on the court.
✓ **Seek professional guidance**: Consult with pickleball equipment experts or professional players to get personalized advice on paddle selection based on your specific needs.
✓ **Test and compare**: Take the time to test different paddles side by side to assess their performance in terms of power, control, touch, and overall feel.
✓ **Consider noise restrictions**: If playing in noise-restricted areas, select a paddle that produces minimal noise upon ball contact.

✓ **Prioritize durability**: Look for paddles made of high-quality materials that can withstand the demands of intense gameplay and last longer.

Remember, choosing the right paddle is a personal decision that depends on your playing style, preferences, and skill level. Take the opportunity to try different paddles, gather information, and make a choice that best suits your needs and enhances your pickleball game. Many sporting goods stores or pickleball clubs offer paddle demo programs, allowing you to test different paddles and find the one that suits you best.

Fast facts:

There is a **sweet spot** in the pickleball paddle. The sweet spot refers to the specific area on the paddle's surface where hitting the ball produces the most optimal combination of power, control, and accuracy. Hitting the ball on the sweet spot results in a cleaner and more efficient shot, maximizing the player's performance. The sweet spot is typically located near the center of the paddle, and players strive to consistently hit the ball in this area for better shot execution.

Understanding paddle regulations and approved specifications

Paddle regulations and approved specifications are essential for both social and competitive pickleball players. The International Federation of Pickleball (IFP) has established guidelines that govern the specifications of pickleball paddles. These regulations ensure fair play, consistency, and a level playing field for all participants.

Paddles must adhere to specific criteria set by the IFP, including length, width, weight, grip circumference, and bounce. These measurements are carefully determined to maintain the integrity of the game and ensure that players have equal opportunities to showcase their skills.

For competitive players, it is crucial to use a paddle that meets the approved specifications. This ensures eligibility to participate in official pickleball tournaments and competitions. Playing with a paddle that does not comply with the regulations can result in disqualification or penalties.

Even for social players who engage in recreational pickleball, understanding paddle regulations can enhance their overall experience. Complying with the specifications ensures that everyone is playing with paddles that are suitable for the game and promotes a consistent and enjoyable playing environment.

To familiarize yourself with the specific paddle regulations and approved specifications, it is recommended to consult the IFP rulebook or reach out to your local pickleball organization. They can provide detailed information on the paddle requirements applicable to your region and offer guidance on choosing a paddle that meets the standards.

By understanding and adhering to paddle regulations and approved specifications, both social and competitive pickleball players can engage in the sport with confidence, fairness, and the assurance that they are playing within the established guidelines.

Top tips:

According to **pickleheads.com**, whether you're a beginner learning to play pickleball or an experienced player looking for the best paddle to improve your game that's as good as you are, it's important to find the one that is right for you. Using the wrong paddle not only affects your play but it can also cost you games. So, finding a blend of power, control, grip, and weight that suits your playing style is key to maximizing your wins.

Pickleheads.com provides reviews of USA Pickleball-approved brands to help you pick the right one for you. They provide reviews and recommendations such as: best paddle, best budget paddle, best for beginners, best intermediate paddle, best advanced paddle, and best under $100.

For example, if you are a **beginner**, and perhaps want a paddle with high-tech performance at an entry level price, you can find out about:

- **characteristics of the paddle** –the paddle weight, length, and width; the handle length; grip circumference; paddle face material; core material; and sweet spot (e.g., large)
- **ratings out of 10** for power, control, spin, and forgiveness
- tips to '**buy if**' (e.g., you've never played pickleball before) and '**pass if**' (e.g., you're intermediate or advanced).

This website also has '**gear guides**' about **balls**, **nets**, **bags**, **shoes**, and **sets**.

This is one of many places to go if you need help making a decision.

2.2   THE BALL: CHOOSING THE RIGHT BOUNCE AND FEEL

When it comes to pickleball, the choice of **ball** (the pickleball ball) can greatly impact the game. The type of ball you use can greatly impact your game, so it is crucial to understand the characteristics and differences between them.
In this section, we will explore the different types of pickleball balls, their characteristics such as bounce and feel, and how to choose the right ball that suits your playing environment and preferences. Understanding the importance of selecting the right ball will ensure a consistent and enjoyable playing experience, whether you're practicing or competing in a game.

Different types of pickleball balls and their attributes (indoor vs. outdoor, ball construction)

A pickleball ball is a unique hollow plastic ball that measures approximately 2.9 inches in diameter and weighs around 0.9 ounces. It features an evenly spaced pattern of 26 to 40 round holes across its surface, which affects its aerodynamics, making it travel slower through the air compared to a solid ball.

These balls are available in various colors such as white, yellow, orange, and green, providing options for players' preferences.

With their durable construction, pickleball balls are designed to withstand the demands of both indoor and outdoor play, making them a versatile choice for players of all levels.

Indoor balls:
Indoor pickleball balls are typically made of a softer material, such as plastic or polymer, and have smaller holes. They are designed to provide better control and slower gameplay, making them ideal for playing on indoor courts with smooth surfaces. The softer material allows for a better grip on the paddle, resulting in enhanced spin and accuracy. Additionally, the smaller holes reduce the ball's speed and bounce, creating a more controlled and strategic game.

Outdoor balls:
Outdoor pickleball balls are built to withstand the elements and the rougher surfaces commonly found on outdoor courts. They are made of a harder plastic material, which increases their durability and resilience to impact. Outdoor balls have larger holes to counteract the wind, as well as to create a faster pace and higher bounce suitable for outdoor play. The increased speed and bounce allow for better performance on outdoor courts with rougher surfaces, ensuring the ball remains playable and easy to track during fast-paced rallies.

Ball construction:
The construction of pickleball balls plays a significant role in their performance and durability. Most balls are made of a durable plastic material, such as polyethylene or PVC, which provides strength and resilience to withstand repeated hits and impacts. The construction affects the ball's weight, bounce, and durability, influencing the overall gameplay experience. High-quality balls are designed to have a consistent bounce and flight pattern, ensuring fairness and predictability during rallies.

The most commonly used ball is the **plastic ball**, which is durable and suitable for outdoor play. **Composite balls** are another popular choice among pickleball players. They are made from a combination of materials, such as plastic and additives like rubber or silica. Composite balls provide a slightly softer feel and are known for their enhanced control, making them a favorite among intermediate and advanced players. These balls are suitable for both indoor and outdoor play.

Selecting the appropriate ball for the playing surface and conditions

Choosing the right ball for the playing surface and conditions is essential for optimal gameplay and enjoyment. Consider the following factors when selecting a pickleball ball:

- **Playing surface**: Determine whether you will be playing on an indoor or outdoor court. Indoor courts typically require softer balls with smaller holes, while outdoor courts necessitate harder balls with larger holes to adapt to rougher surfaces and wind conditions.
- **Court type**: Consider the type of court surface you will be playing on, such as concrete, asphalt, or a specially designed pickleball court surface. Different surfaces may affect the ball's bounce and behavior, so choose a ball that is suitable for the specific court type.
- **Climate**: Take into account the weather conditions in which you will be playing. If you frequently play in hot or humid climates, choose balls that are designed to withstand high temperatures and maintain their performance. Similarly, if you often play in colder conditions, look for balls that remain responsive and have consistent bounce even in lower temperatures.
- **Skill level:** Consider your skill level and that of your fellow players. Beginners may benefit from using balls with slower speeds and more control, allowing for longer rallies and improved shot placement. Advanced players may prefer balls with faster speeds and higher bounce to challenge their skills and facilitate faster-paced gameplay.

The choice of ball can affect factors such as speed, bounce, and spin, thereby impacting your strategy and overall gameplay. It is advisable to try out different balls and see which one suits your playing style and preferences.

Exploring the importance of ball consistency and durability

In pickleball, **ball consistency** and **durability** play a crucial role in the overall playing experience. Let's delve deeper into the importance of these two factors:

Ball consistency:
Consistency refers to the uniformity of the ball's performance characteristics, such as bounce height, flight pattern, and responsiveness. When a ball is consistent, players can rely on its behavior and make accurate judgments during gameplay. Here's why ball consistency matters:

- **Predictability**: Consistent bounce and flight patterns allow players to anticipate how the ball will behave, enabling them to position themselves effectively and execute shots with precision.
- **Skill development**: Consistent balls provide a reliable platform for players to develop their skills and strategies. With consistent performance, players can practice and refine their techniques, ultimately improving their overall game.
- **Fairness**: In both recreational and competitive play, consistent balls ensure fairness among players. When everyone is playing with the same predictable ball characteristics, the game becomes more balanced and competitive.

Ball durability:
Durability refers to the ball's ability to withstand the rigors of gameplay and maintain its performance over time. Here's why ball durability is important:

- **Longevity**: Durable balls have a longer lifespan, allowing for extended use and minimizing the need for frequent replacements. This not only saves costs but also ensures a consistent playing experience over an extended period.
- **Cost-effectiveness**: By investing in durable balls, players can avoid constantly purchasing new ones. Durable balls are built to withstand hard hits, impacts, and varying weather conditions, providing excellent value for money.
- **Reliable performance**: A durable ball maintains its shape, bounce, and flight characteristics throughout its lifespan. This ensures that players can rely on consistent performance and enjoy a satisfying game every time they step onto the court.

Consistent balls allow players to anticipate and react effectively, fostering skill development and fair play. Meanwhile, durable balls provide long-lasting performance, saving costs and ensuring a reliable playing experience. By recognizing the significance of ball consistency and durability, players can make informed choices when selecting balls, leading to enhanced enjoyment and success on the pickleball court.

If you're just getting into pickleball, you might not care too much about the ball. However, if you start playing competitively, tournaments have requirements on what balls to use; so, specific brands may become important.

Fast facts:

As you progress in your pickleball journey, it is crucial to consider the regulations and guidelines set by governing bodies such as the USA Pickleball Association (USAPA). They provide specific requirements for tournament play, including the approved ball types and specifications.

10 top tips for choosing the right pickleball ball for you

Here are the top pieces of advice for choosing the right pickleball ball:

1. **Consider your skill level**: Whether you're a novice or an experienced player, select a ball that matches your skill level. Beginners may benefit from balls with a slightly softer feel, while advanced players might prefer balls with a livelier bounce.
2. **Determine the playing surface**: Different pickleball balls are designed for specific playing surfaces, such as indoor or outdoor courts. Choose a ball that is suitable for the type of court you'll be playing on.
3. **Assess ball durability**: Look for balls made with durable materials that can withstand the rigors of regular gameplay. Opt for balls that are known for their longevity and resistance to cracking or splitting.

4. **Evaluate ball consistency**: Consistency in bounce and flight characteristics is essential for a fair and enjoyable game. Select balls that offer consistent performance to ensure a level playing field.
5. **Consider noise level**: Some pickleball balls produce more noise upon impact than others. If noise is a concern, choose balls that are designed to minimize sound, especially if you'll be playing in noise-sensitive areas.
6. **Test different brands**: Try out different brands and models of pickleball balls to find the one that suits your personal preference. Each brand may offer slight variations in terms of feel, bounce, and playability.
7. **Seek recommendations**: Ask for recommendations from fellow pickleball players, coaches, or local pickleball communities. They can provide insights and suggestions based on their experiences with different balls.
8. **Check ball approval**: Look for balls that are approved by pickleball governing bodies, such as the International Federation of Pickleball (IFP). Approved balls meet specific standards for size, weight, and bounce.
9. **Consider visibility**: Opt for balls with high visibility colors, such as neon or vibrant shades, to enhance visibility and make it easier to track the ball during gameplay, especially in low-light conditions.
10. **Balance performance and price**: While it's important to invest in quality pickleball balls, consider your budget. Find a ball that offers good performance and durability within your price range.

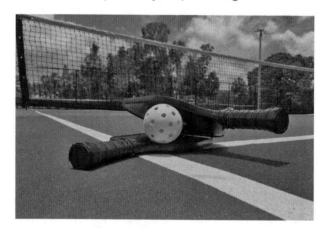

2.3   DRESSING THE PART: PERFORMANCE AND STYLE ON THE COURT

Dressing for success on the pickleball court goes beyond just looking good—it's about optimizing your performance and comfort. Choosing the right clothing can make a world of difference in your game, allowing you to move freely, stay cool, and focus on your shots. From moisture-wicking fabrics to strategic ventilation, the right apparel can help you stay comfortable, dry, and confident throughout your matches.

Recommended clothing for pickleball, considering comfort and mobility

When it comes to choosing clothing for pickleball, it's important to prioritize comfort and mobility. Here are some recommendations:

- **Opt for breathable fabrics**: Choose clothing made from breathable materials such as polyester or nylon. These fabrics allow air to circulate and help wick away sweat, keeping you cool and comfortable during gameplay.
- **Moisture-wicking technology**: Look for clothing with moisture-wicking properties. This technology helps to pull sweat away from your skin, keeping you dry and preventing discomfort caused by dampness.
- **Consider lightweight and stretchy materials**: Pick clothing that is lightweight and offers ample stretch. This allows for unrestricted movement on the court and enhances your range of motion during shots and quick direction changes.
- **Choose comfortable fit**: Select clothing that provides a comfortable fit. Avoid garments that are too tight or restrictive, as they may hinder your movement. Opt for a relaxed fit that allows for ease of movement without excess fabric that could get in the way.
- **Protection from the sun**: If playing outdoors, consider clothing with built-in sun protection, such as UPF-rated fabrics. This helps shield your skin from harmful UV rays and reduces the risk of sunburn.

Importance of moisture-wicking fabrics and breathable materials

Moisture-wicking fabrics and breathable materials play a vital role in enhancing comfort and performance during pickleball. Here's why they are important:

- **Moisture management**: Pickleball can be a physically demanding sport, causing you to sweat. **Moisture-wicking fabrics** pull sweat away from your skin and onto the surface of the fabric, where it evaporates more quickly. This helps regulate your body temperature and prevents excessive sweating, discomfort, and chafing.
- **Quick drying**: Moisture-wicking fabrics have the ability to dry quickly, which is beneficial during intense gameplay or when playing in hot and humid conditions. By keeping you dry, these fabrics help maintain your body's optimal temperature and prevent overheating.
- **Breathability**: Breathable materials allow air to flow through the fabric, promoting ventilation and heat dissipation. This helps to keep you cool and comfortable during long matches or in warm climates. It also prevents the buildup of moisture and odor, ensuring a fresh and pleasant playing experience.
- **Strategic ventilation**: This means having breathable parts in clothing to let air in and sweat out. In pickleball, it's important to have clothing with **strategic ventilation**, like mesh or perforated panels, in places where you get hot and sweaty. This helps keep you cool and comfortable while playing. It allows air to circulate and removes excess heat and moisture, so you can stay focused on the game.

Guidelines for appropriate attire and dress codes in various settings

While pickleball is often played in a casual and recreational setting, it's important to be aware of any specific dress codes or guidelines that may be in place, particularly in organized events or certain facilities. Here are some general guidelines to keep in mind:

- **Respect the venue**: Some pickleball facilities or clubs may have specific dress codes, particularly if they are affiliated with other sports or have certain standards in place. Respect any rules regarding attire and ensure you adhere to them.
- **Appropriate coverage**: Choose clothing that provides appropriate coverage. Avoid overly revealing or offensive attire that may be deemed inappropriate for a family-friendly environment.
- **Non-marking shoes**: Many pickleball facilities require non-marking shoes to protect the court surface. Check with the facility or organizers to ensure you have the appropriate footwear.
- **Consideration for others**: Keep in mind that while comfort and mobility are important, it's also important to consider the comfort of others. Avoid wearing clothing with distracting graphics or slogans that may disrupt gameplay or cause distractions.

By following these guidelines and choosing appropriate attire, you can ensure a comfortable and respectful playing experience for yourself and those around you.

2.4   FOOTWEAR: FINDING THE PERFECT FIT FOR AGILITY AND SUPPORT

Finding the perfect pair of shoes is essential for enhancing your agility, stability, and overall performance on the court. Here, we will explore the importance of proper footwear and guide you through the process of selecting the right shoes that provide both comfort and support. Whether you're a beginner or a seasoned player, having the right footwear can make a significant difference in your game.

Importance of proper footwear for pickleball, focusing on stability and traction

Proper footwear is crucial for pickleball as it provides the necessary stability and traction to support your movements on the court. Here's why it's important:

- **Enhanced stability**: Pickleball involves quick lateral movements, pivoting, and changes in direction. The right footwear with proper stability features, such as reinforced sidewalls and supportive midsoles, helps prevent excessive ankle rolling and provides a stable base for your movements.
- **Reliable traction**: The court surface in pickleball can vary, from indoor courts with smooth surfaces to outdoor courts with different textures. Shoes with a specialized outsole design, featuring multi-directional treads or herringbone patterns, offer excellent traction, allowing you to grip the court and make quick, precise movements.

- **Impact absorption**: Although the sport is relatively low impact, some of the repetitive movements in pickleball, such as jumping and lunging, can put stress on your joints. Properly cushioned shoes with shock-absorbing midsoles help reduce the impact on your feet, ankles, knees, and hips, minimizing the risk of injuries like sprains or stress fractures.

Characteristics of pickleball shoes and considerations for different court surfaces

When selecting pickleball shoes, keep the following characteristics and court surface considerations in mind:

- **Court-specific design**: Pickleball shoes are designed specifically for the sport, with features that optimize performance on the court. Look for shoes labeled as pickleball-specific or suitable for multi-court sports.
- **Cushioning and support**: Choose shoes with adequate cushioning and support to minimize the impact on your joints and provide comfort during extended play. Look for features like padded insoles, cushioned midsoles, and supportive ankle collars.
- **Durability and breathability:** Pickleball shoes should be durable enough to withstand the demands of the sport. Look for materials that offer durability, such as synthetic leather or reinforced mesh. Additionally, choose shoes with breathable uppers to keep your feet cool and comfortable.
- **Court surface considerations**: Consider the type of court surface you will be playing on. Indoor courts typically have smoother surfaces, so shoes with a non-marking outsole and a good grip are essential. Outdoor courts may have a rougher texture, so shoes with more aggressive tread patterns provide better traction.

Tips for selecting the right shoe size and fit for optimal performance and injury prevention

To ensure optimal performance and minimize the risk of injuries, follow these **tips** when selecting the right shoe size and fit:

- ✓ **Measure your feet**: Have your feet measured professionally to determine your accurate shoe size. Remember that foot size can change over time, so measure both feet and choose the size that accommodates the larger foot.
- ✓ **Allow room for toe movement**: There should be a thumb's width of space between your longest toe and the end of the shoe. This allows for natural movement and prevents cramped toes during intense gameplay.
- ✓ **Snug heel fit**: The heel should fit snugly, with minimal slippage. A secure heel fit prevents your foot from sliding within the shoe and provides stability during lateral movements.
- ✓ **Try shoes with socks**: When trying on pickleball shoes, wear the same type of socks you would typically wear during gameplay. This ensures a more accurate fit and prevents any discomfort caused by mismatched sizing.
- ✓ **Walk and test**: Walk and move around in the shoes to assess their comfort, support, and overall fit. Pay attention to any pressure points or areas of discomfort that may indicate an improper fit.

2.5   OTHER EQUIPMENT AND ACCESSORIES

In addition to the basic equipment, there are other accessories and items that can enhance the pickleball experience.

- Many players choose to use grip enhancers, such as **overgrips** or **grip tapes**, to improve paddle grip and prevent slipping during play.
- **Paddle covers** are useful for protecting the paddle face from scratches and damage during transport or storage. Some players opt for **paddle edge guards** to provide added protection to the edges of the paddle.
- Accessories like wristbands or headbands can help absorb sweat and keep hands and forehead dry.
- Pickleball **gloves** are gloves worn by pickleball players to improve their grip on the paddle, keep their hands warm in cold weather, or reduce sweaty hands. They are designed to absorb moisture while allowing air to pass through, which helps to improve the game and strengthen the grip over the paddle. They can be made from a variety of materials, including leather, synthetic leather, and other breathable fabrics.
- Water bottles are essential to stay hydrated during gameplay.
- It's also advisable to have a towel handy for wiping off perspiration or the ball.
- Pickleball bags or backpacks designed specifically for carrying paddles, balls, and other equipment are convenient for transporting gear to and from the court.
- Additionally, players may consider investing in sunglasses with UV protection and hats or visors to shield the eyes and face from the sun's glare and heat.

Fast facts:

In pickleball doubles, the **first server band** is a form of identification worn by the player who serves first for their team. It is typically a wristband or other visible marker that helps players keep track of who served first and avoid confusion during the game. The first server band can be especially helpful in remembering the server rotation and avoiding disputes over who should be serving. For example, if a long rally occurs and players forget who served the ball, they can look for the player wearing the first server band to help determine who should serve next. The first server band is not a requirement, but it can be a useful tool to help keep the game running smoothly!

Pickleball kits for beginners?

As a beginning pickleball player, you might be wondering whether it's better to purchase a pickleball kit or buy the items individually.

A **pickleball kit** is a package or set that includes various items needed to play the sport. A typical pickleball kit may contain paddles, balls, a portable pickleball net, and other accessories, such as a carrying bag or case.

The purpose of a pickleball kit is to provide beginners with the basic equipment necessary to start playing pickleball. It offers a convenient and cost-effective option for those who want to get started without the hassle of purchasing individual items separately. By providing all the essential components in one package, pickleball kits make it easier for beginners to get on the court and enjoy the game right away.

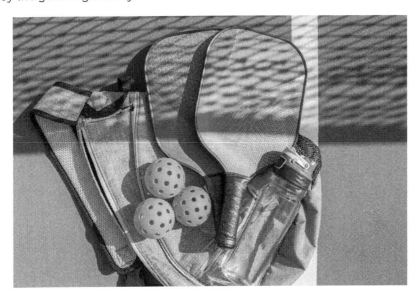

Here are a few factors to consider:

- **Convenience**: Purchasing a pickleball kit can be a convenient option, especially if you're starting from scratch and don't have any equipment. Kits typically include everything you need to get started, such as paddles, balls, and a net. This saves you time and effort in searching for individual items.
- **Cost**: Kits often provide a cost-effective solution, as they bundle multiple items together at a lower price compared to buying them individually. If you're on a budget and looking to get all the necessary equipment in one go, a kit might be a more affordable choice.
- **Customization**: On the other hand, buying items individually allows for more customization. You have the flexibility to choose paddles and balls that suit your preferences, whether it's based on grip size, weight, or specific features. This approach gives you more control over tailoring the equipment to your playing style.
- **Quality and performance**: Individual purchases often allow for more research and comparison shopping, which can lead to selecting higher-quality items based on personal reviews and recommendations. While kits may provide basic equipment, investing in higher-quality paddles and balls individually can enhance your performance and enjoyment on the court.

It's important to make sure that the set you choose includes high-quality equipment from reputable brands. If you're not sure about the quality of the equipment in a starter set, or if you have specific preferences for your equipment, you might consider purchasing items individually to ensure that you get exactly what you want.

Ultimately, the decision between purchasing a kit or buying items individually depends on your specific needs, preferences, and budget. If you're looking for convenience and a cost-effective solution, a pickleball kit might be a good starting point. However, if you prioritize customization and quality, purchasing items individually allows for more personalized choices. Consider your priorities and assess the available options to make the best decision for your pickleball journey.

By selecting the appropriate equipment and accessories, players can optimize their performance, comfort, and enjoyment of the game of pickleball.

Top tips:

When choosing **pickleball equipment**, it's important to consider your skill level, playing style, and personal preferences. Take the time to research different brands and products, read reviews, and compare features and prices. If possible, try out the equipment before making a purchase to ensure that it feels comfortable and performs well. Remember that investing in high-quality equipment can enhance your playing experience and help you improve your game.

2.6   EQUIPMENT MAINTENANCE: CARING FOR YOUR GEAR

It is important to understand the significance of equipment care and maintenance to enhance your overall playing experience. Proper care and maintenance not only prolong the lifespan of your gear but also ensure that you are playing with equipment that is in optimal condition. Here are some tips:

Paddles:

Your paddle is your most important piece of equipment, and it requires regular care.

✓ Keep your paddle clean by wiping it down with a damp cloth after each use.
✓ Avoid excessive exposure to sunlight and moisture, as it can damage the paddle's surface.
✓ Store your paddle in a protective cover or case to prevent scratches and dings.
✓ Check the grip regularly and replace it if it shows signs of wear or becomes slippery.
✓ Avoid dropping or banging the paddle against hard surfaces to prevent damage.

Pickleballs:

Pickleballs can wear out over time due to constant use. Inspect balls regularly for cracks, dents, or other signs of damage.

- ✓ Store pickleball balls in a cool and dry place to maintain their quality.
- ✓ Avoid leaving them exposed to extreme temperatures or direct sunlight, as this can affect their performance.
- ✓ Clean dirty balls using mild soap and water and dry them thoroughly before storing.
- ✓ Inspect the balls for cracks, dents, or deformities and replace them if necessary.
- ✓ Avoid using worn-out or damaged balls during play to ensure consistent bounce and performance. If a ball is no longer round or has lost its bounce, it's time to replace it.
- ✓ Rotate your balls periodically to distribute the wear evenly.

Nets and posts:

If you have a personal net and posts, make sure to inspect them regularly.

- ✓ Regularly check the net tension and adjust it if needed to ensure proper height and tightness.
- ✓ Clean the net with a soft brush or cloth to remove dirt and debris.
- ✓ Inspect the net and posts for any signs of damage or wear, such as fraying or rust.
- ✓ Replace worn-out or damaged parts promptly to maintain the integrity of the net system.
- ✓ Store the net and posts in a dry place when not in use to prevent rust and deterioration.

Shoes:

Investing in a good pair of court shoes is crucial for your comfort and safety.

- ✓ Clean your pickleball shoes regularly by wiping off dirt and debris.
- ✓ Allow your shoes to air dry after each use to prevent odor and moisture buildup.
- ✓ Avoid exposing your shoes to extreme heat or direct sunlight, as it can damage the materials.
- ✓ Rotate between multiple pairs of shoes to extend their lifespan and allow them to dry between uses.
- ✓ Replace your shoes when the outsole is worn, cushioning is compressed, or there is a noticeable decline in support.

CHAPTER 3   MASTERING THE BASICS

Welcome to **Chapter 3**. In this chapter, we will explore the essential skills and techniques that form the foundation of a strong pickleball game. From mastering the grip for control and spin to understanding the importance of the ready position, we will delve into the intricacies of upper body techniques and the fundamental footwork principles. Whether you're a beginner looking to establish a solid foundation or an experienced player aiming to refine your skills, this chapter will provide you with the knowledge and guidance to elevate your pickleball game to new heights. Get ready to hone your skills, improve your technique, and unleash your full potential on the court.

3.1   GRIP LIKE A PRO: CONTROL AND SPIN UNLEASHED

Different grip styles in pickleball (eastern grip, continental grip, and western grip)

In pickleball, the grip you use on your paddle plays a crucial role in controlling your shots and executing different techniques. Here are the **three main grip styles** used in pickleball:

Eastern grip:

The **eastern grip** is the most popular paddle grip in pickleball and is generally recommended for beginner and intermediate players. It is a universal or neutral grip that allows you to hit both forehand and backhand shots with the same grip. It is considered the perfect compromise between a forehand and backhand shot. To find this Eastern pickleball grip, hold your pickleball paddle directly out in front of you with your opposite hand, such that the paddle face is looking evenly to the left of your body and to the right of your body. Take your hand that you are holding the pickleball paddle with and place it on the face of the pickleball paddle. Slide your hand down the paddle face and shake hands with the pickleball paddle grip.

Continental grip:

The **continental grip** is also considered a "neutral" grip because it is relatively easy to use for both forehand and backhand shots. It is not particularly strong for either shot, but it is versatile and can be used for a variety of shots, including dinks, volleys, and topspin forehands. To find this grip, place your hand flat against the face of the racket (paddle), then slide your hand down to the grip. Your index knuckle and the heel of your hand should be on the second bevel of the grip.

Western grip:

The **western grip** produces a lot of topspin but makes it more difficult to hit backhand shots. It causes your palm to be generally behind the paddle on a forehand, which results in powerful forehands. However, it is not recommended for beginners as it can make hitting backhands more difficult. To find this

Western pickleball grip, start in an Eastern grip and turn your wrist 90 degrees clockwise for righties, or 90 degrees counterclockwise for lefties.

Each grip has its own advantages and disadvantages and can be used for specific shots or changed during play.

As a beginner to pickleball, it is generally recommended to start with the **eastern grip**. As you progress in the game and develop your skills, you may want to experiment with different grips to find what works best for your playing style and preferred shots. Some players may prefer to stick with one grip throughout the game, while others may change grips depending on the shot they are hitting.

It's important to experiment with different grips to find what works best for your playing style and preferred shots.

Whether or not you should change grips during a match depends on your personal preferences and playing style. Some players may prefer to stick with one grip throughout the game, while others may change grips depending on the shot they are hitting. It's important to experiment and find what works best for you.

Proper hand placement and technique for optimal control and shot variety

Proper hand placement and technique are essential for achieving optimal control and shot variety in pickleball. Follow these guidelines for hand placement and technique:

- **Hand position**: Place your hand on the paddle handle with a firm but relaxed grip. Ensure that your fingers wrap around the handle comfortably, allowing for flexibility and maneuverability.
- **Balance and stability**: Maintain a balanced and stable grip by keeping your wrist firm and neutral. Avoid excessive wrist movement, as it can lead to inconsistent shots.
- **Ready position**: Position your hand slightly towards the end of the handle for better maneuverability and reaction time. This ready position allows for quick adjustments and faster shot execution.
- **Shot execution**: Maintain a loose grip during your stroke and contact with the ball. This allows for better feel and control of the paddle, resulting in more accurate shots.

Importance of grip pressure and adjusting it based on shot requirements

Grip pressure is an important aspect of pickleball technique that affects shot control and power. Consider the following points regarding grip pressure:

- **Control and accuracy**: Proper grip pressure allows for better control and accuracy of your shots. A firm but relaxed grip helps maintain stability while allowing for a smooth swing and follow-through.

- **Shot variation**: Adjusting grip pressure enables you to vary the speed and spin of your shots. A lighter grip can generate more power and spin, while a firmer grip provides more control and accuracy.
- **Adaptation to shot requirements**: Modify your grip pressure based on the specific shot requirements. For delicate shots like dinks or soft drops, a lighter grip with gentle touch is necessary. For powerful drives or smashes, a firmer grip with increased pressure is needed.
- **Avoid excessive grip pressure**: Be mindful not to over-grip the paddle, as it can lead to tension in your hand, arm, and shoulder muscles, affecting your stroke fluidity and causing fatigue.

Top tips:

What are some **common mistakes beginners make** about the **grip** and what are some **tips to remedy** them?

Gripping the paddle too tightly: Many beginners tend to hold the paddle with a tight grip, which can limit wrist flexibility and hinder shot control. **Remedy**: Practice holding the paddle with a relaxed but firm grip. Find a balance where you can have control without unnecessary tension in your hand.

Holding the paddle too low or too high: Beginners may struggle with finding the optimal hand position on the grip. Holding the paddle too low can limit reach and power, while holding it too high can reduce control. **Remedy**: Position your hand on the grip at a comfortable mid-point, allowing for a balanced and versatile stroke.

Incorrect finger positioning: Beginners may inadvertently place their fingers in improper positions on the paddle grip, affecting stability and control. **Remedy**: Ensure your fingers are spread comfortably across the grip, providing balance and stability. Avoid gripping the paddle solely with your fingertips or clenching it with all your fingers tightly together.

Inconsistent grip pressure: Maintaining consistent grip pressure throughout the swing is crucial for accurate shots. Beginners may unintentionally apply varying levels of pressure during their strokes, leading to inconsistent results. **Remedy**: Focus on maintaining a steady grip pressure throughout the swing, avoiding sudden changes that can affect shot accuracy.

Failure to adjust grip for different shots: Beginners sometimes overlook the importance of adjusting their grip for different types of shots. Using the same grip for all shots can limit control and power. **Remedy**: Practice adapting your grip to different shots. Experiment with softer grips for delicate shots like dinks and volleys, and firmer grips for more powerful shots such as drives and smashes.

By addressing these common grip mistakes and implementing the suggested remedies, beginners can improve their overall control, power, and consistency in pickleball. Remember to practice regularly and seek feedback from experienced players or coaches to fine-tune your grip technique.

By understanding and utilizing different grip styles, maintaining proper hand placement and technique, and adjusting grip pressure as needed, you can achieve better control, shot variety, and overall performance in pickleball. Experiment with different grips and find the one that suits your playing style and shot preferences.

3.2   READY POSITION: A LAUNCHPAD FOR QUICK REACTIONS

The **ready position** is a proactive stance that allows players to anticipate and react to incoming shots with ease. It helps players maintain balance, control, and agility on the court, ensuring they are prepared for any shot that comes their way. Adopting the ready position as a foundational element of your game can greatly enhance your ability to move swiftly, react effectively, and execute shots with precision in pickleball.

Explanation of the ready position and its role in maintaining balance and readiness

The ready position is a fundamental stance in pickleball that allows players to maintain balance and readiness for quick movement and shot execution. It refers to a specific body and paddle position that prepares players to react effectively to their opponent's shots. Here's an explanation of the ready position and its importance:

✓ **Body position**: Stand with your feet shoulder-width apart, knees slightly bent, and weight evenly distributed between both feet. This balanced stance provides stability and allows for quick changes in direction.
✓ **Paddle position**: Hold your paddle with both hands in front of you, parallel to the ground and slightly below waist level. Keep your elbows comfortably bent and close to your body. This position allows for quick reactions and easy paddle maneuverability.
✓ **Readiness**: The ready position puts you in a state of readiness to respond to your opponent's shots.

By being in this position, you can react quickly and efficiently to retrieve shots and maintain control of the game.

Proper stance and body positioning for quick movement and efficient shot execution

A proper stance and body positioning are essential for maximizing your movement and executing shots efficiently in pickleball.

Here's what you need to know:

✓ **Footwork**: Keep your feet positioned slightly wider than shoulder-width apart to provide a stable base. This allows for better lateral and forward/backward movement.

✓ **Weight distribution**: Distribute your weight evenly on both feet, avoiding excessive weight on the heels or toes. This balanced weight distribution allows for quick weight shifts and agile movements.

✓ **Body alignment**: Align your body with the net and the direction you want to move. Face the net with your shoulders squared, hips facing forward, and torso slightly leaning forward. This position optimizes your ability to move swiftly in any direction.

Top tips:

What are some **common mistakes beginners make** about the **ready position** and what are some **tips to remedy** them?

Standing too upright: One common mistake is standing too upright in the ready position, which can limit mobility and reaction time. **Remedy**: Bend your knees slightly, keeping a comfortable athletic stance. This helps with balance, quick movements, and the ability to react to incoming shots.

Holding the paddle too high or too low: Beginners may hold the paddle either too high or too low in the ready position, affecting their reach and readiness to respond. **Remedy**: Position the paddle at a mid-level, around waist height, allowing for quick and efficient paddle movement and easy access to both forehand and backhand shots.

Gripping the paddle too tightly: Holding the paddle with a tight grip in the ready position can lead to unnecessary tension and slow reaction time. **Remedy**: Maintain a relaxed and loose grip on the paddle, promoting quick adjustments and fluid movement during play.

Lack of active footwork: Beginners may have a tendency to keep their feet stationary in the ready position, which limits their ability to move quickly and efficiently. **Remedy**: Stay light on your feet, maintaining small, quick steps, and being ready to move in any direction. This allows for better court coverage and the ability to reach shots effectively.

Poor body alignment: Beginners may have difficulty aligning their body properly in the ready position, which can lead to decreased stability and limited shot options. **Remedy**: Face the net squarely, with your shoulders parallel to the net, ensuring a balanced and stable position to react to shots from all angles.

By addressing these common mistakes and implementing the suggested remedies, beginners can improve their readiness, mobility, and overall performance on the pickleball court. Remember to practice the proper ready position regularly and focus on staying alert and prepared for every shot.

The importance of staying on the balls of the feet and being light on the toes

Staying on the balls of your feet and being light on your toes is crucial for maintaining agility and responsiveness on the pickleball court. Here's why it matters:

- **Quick movement**: Being on the balls of your feet allows for quicker and more explosive movement. It enables you to react swiftly to shots and cover the court effectively.
- **Balance and stability**: By staying light on your toes, you maintain better balance and stability. This helps you maintain a ready position and respond to shots with control and precision.
- **Improved court coverage**: Being light on your toes facilitates quick weight transfers and allows you to move in any direction efficiently. It enhances your court coverage and enables you to reach shots effectively.
- **Quicker shot execution**: Being on the balls of your feet allows for faster weight shifts, enabling you to execute shots with speed and accuracy. It also facilitates swift recovery to a ready position after each shot.

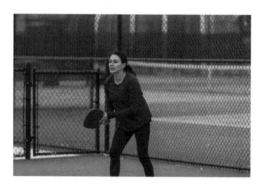

Maintaining the ready position, adopting a proper stance and body positioning, and staying on the balls of your feet are key elements in maximizing your movement, shot execution, and overall performance in pickleball. Practice these techniques to improve your agility, balance, and responsiveness on the court.

3.3   SWING WITH PRECISION: MASTERING UPPER BODY TECHNIQUES

In the game of pickleball, mastering the **upper body techniques** is crucial for achieving precision, control, and power in your shots. The upper body mechanics encompass the coordinated movements of your arms, shoulders, and core, which are fundamental to executing different shots effectively. This section will delve into the intricacies of the upper body mechanics and guide you through exploring various shot types, refining techniques, and improving overall shot execution.

Understanding the upper body mechanics in pickleball shots

To excel in pickleball, it is essential to have a solid understanding of the **upper body mechanics** involved in different shots. Upper-body mechanics refers to the movements and actions performed by the upper body, including the arms, shoulders, and torso, during pickleball. It encompasses techniques and motions involved in striking the ball, such as the swing, follow-through, and coordination of the upper body to generate power, control, and accuracy in shots.

This section will break down the key elements to help you develop a strong foundation for your game.

- **Grip and hand placement**: Start by mastering the grip and hand placement on the paddle. The most common grip in pickleball is the continental grip, where the base knuckle of your index finger rests on the slanted part of the paddle. This grip allows for versatility in executing various shots.
- **Ready position**: The ready position is the foundation for every shot in pickleball. Stand with your feet shoulder-width apart, knees slightly bent, and weight evenly distributed. Keep your paddle up and in front of you, maintaining a relaxed but alert posture. The ready position allows for quick reactions and efficient shot execution.
- **Upper body alignment**: Maintaining proper upper body alignment is essential for generating power and accuracy in your shots. Align your shoulders, hips, and feet towards the target or desired shot direction. This alignment helps transfer energy effectively and improves shot consistency.

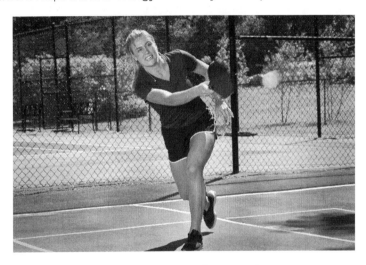

Exploring different types of shots and their execution

Pickleball offers a variety of **shots** that players can use to strategically outmaneuver their opponents. Understanding the different types of shots and their execution is vital for developing a versatile and effective game. Let's delve deeper into each shot type and explore some valuable tips for executing them with finesse.

Serve:
Understanding the different serving techniques is crucial to mastering the game. The **serve** is the first shot you make in each rally, and it sets the tone for the entire point.

The **serve** is the starting shot in pickleball, setting the tone for the rally. Here are some tips to improve your serve:

- ✓ **Focus on a consistent toss**: Practice a reliable release or drop that allows you to make clean contact with the ball at the desired height.
- ✓ **Maintain a relaxed grip**: Avoid excessive tension in your grip to promote a smooth and controlled swing.
- ✓ **Use your legs**: Engage your legs and transfer your weight from back to front as you swing, generating power and accuracy.
- ✓ **Aim for strategic placement**: Experiment with different serve placements to keep your opponent off balance and exploit their weaknesses.

Groundstrokes:

Groundstrokes refer to shots hit after the ball has bounced. Mastering groundstrokes involves proper footwork, timing, and coordination. Consider these tips for effective groundstroke execution:

- ✓ **Establish a solid base**: Position yourself with a wide stance and bend your knees to provide stability and balance.
- ✓ **Maintain a relaxed grip**: Avoid gripping the paddle too tightly, as it can restrict your swing motion. Opt for a loose and controlled grip.
- ✓ **Rotate your body**: Initiate the shot by rotating your shoulders and hips towards the desired target, generating power and enabling proper stroke mechanics.
- ✓ **Aim for consistency and placement**: Focus on consistent contact with the ball and strive to place your groundstrokes strategically to keep your opponent on the move.

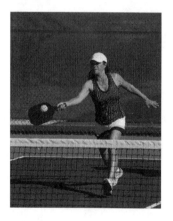
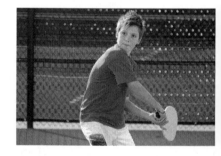

Volleys:

Volleys are shots played in the air before the ball bounces. They require quick reflexes and precise hand-eye coordination. Consider these tips for executing effective volleys:

- ✓ **Get into proper position**: Position yourself near the Non-Volley Zone (kitchen) to be ready for volleys. Bend your knees and stay light on your feet to react quickly.
- ✓ **Use short and compact swings**: Keep your volleys concise and controlled, using short backswings and quick forward motions.

✓ **Focus on soft hands:** Maintain a gentle grip and use your wrists to absorb the pace of the incoming ball, directing it with finesse.
✓ **Aim for placement and angle**: Look for opportunities to place your volleys away from your opponent's reach, creating difficult returns.

Dinks:

Dinks are soft shots played close to the net, aimed at placing the ball in hard-to-reach areas for your opponent. Here are some tips to improve your dinking skills:

✓ **Use a continental grip**: Adopt a continental grip for better control and maneuverability in executing dinks.
✓ **Short and compact swing**: Keep your swing short and controlled, focusing on touch rather than power.
✓ **Employ soft hands and light touch**: Apply minimal force to the ball, aiming for a soft, delicate shot that drops close to the net.
✓ **Vary your placement and angles**: Mix up your dinks by placing them in different areas of the opponent's court, making it challenging for them to anticipate your shots.

By understanding the nuances of each shot type and implementing these tips, you will enhance your shot execution in pickleball. Remember to practice regularly and incorporate these techniques into your game to develop a well-rounded skill set and keep your opponents guessing.

Fast facts:

Shots and strokes? In pickleball, it's important to understand the distinction between shots and strokes. While the terms are often used interchangeably, they refer to different aspects of gameplay.

Shots in pickleball are the specific types of shots or techniques used to play the ball, such as the lob, dink, drive, or drop shot. These shots describe the intended trajectory, speed, and placement of the ball.

On the other hand, **strokes** refer to the technique or motion used to execute those shots. Strokes encompass the mechanics and body movements involved in hitting the ball with the paddle, including the forehand stroke, backhand stroke, and serving motion. For example, the forehand stroke can be used to execute various shots like a forehand drive, forehand lob, or forehand drop shot.

By understanding the difference between shots and strokes, players can develop a repertoire of shots and refine their stroke mechanics to enhance their overall performance on the pickleball court.

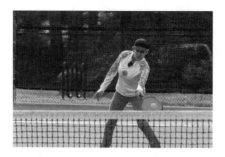

Refining upper body techniques for precision and control

To achieve precision and control in your pickleball shots, it is essential to refine your upper body techniques. This section will provide valuable insights into how you can improve your shot-making abilities.

✓ **Follow-through**: Ensure a complete follow-through after each shot. Let your swing continue naturally even after contact with the ball, maintaining a smooth and fluid motion. A proper follow-through helps with shot accuracy and control.
✓ **Weight transfer**: Shift your weight from your back foot to your front foot during the shot to generate power and maintain balance. The transfer of weight adds momentum to your swing and improves shot stability.
✓ **Timing and rhythm**: Develop a sense of timing and rhythm by practicing your shots consistently. Pay attention to the ball's trajectory and timing your swing to meet the ball at the optimal point. This synchronization enhances your shot-making capabilities.

3.4   FOOTWORK FUNDAMENTALS: LIGHT ON YOUR FEET

Effective footwork is a critical aspect of pickleball, allowing players to move swiftly, maintain balance, and position themselves optimally on the court. In this section, we will delve into the footwork fundamentals that will help you improve your agility, court coverage, and shot execution. We will explore footwork patterns for different shots, techniques for efficient movement and positioning, and strategies for anticipating and reacting to opponents' shots.

Exploring the footwork patterns for different shots (sideways shuffle, split step, crossover step, cross step)

Different shots in pickleball require specific footwork patterns to enable quick movements and proper positioning. Let's examine four essential footwork patterns:

Sideways shuffle:

The **sideways shuffle** is a crucial footwork technique in pickleball that allows players to move laterally across the court with speed and agility. To execute the sideways shuffle correctly, start with your feet shoulder-width apart and slightly bend your knees. Keeping your weight centered and your body low, shuffle your feet quickly and smoothly in small steps, moving laterally from side to side.

This technique enables you to cover ground efficiently and maintain proper positioning, ensuring that you can quickly react to shots played towards the sides of the court. Whether you need to defend against wide shots or reach for balls hit towards the sidelines, the sideways shuffle allows you to move swiftly and maintain good court coverage, setting you up for effective shots or successful defensive plays.

Split step:

The **split step** is a fundamental footwork technique in pickleball that helps players prepare for an incoming shot and react quickly to their opponent's movement. To execute the split step correctly, stand with your feet shoulder-width apart and slightly bend your knees. As your opponent makes contact with the ball, jump lightly off the ground, bringing your feet together in mid-air, and then land softly with your weight evenly distributed.

The split step allows you to be ready and balanced, improving your reaction time and enabling quick movements in any direction. It is particularly important when anticipating your opponent's shots, allowing you to adjust your positioning and respond effectively. The split step is a versatile footwork technique that helps you stay in control and quickly adapt to the changing dynamics of the game.

Crossover step:

The **crossover step** is a footwork technique used to change direction quickly and efficiently on the pickleball court. To perform the crossover step, start with your feet shoulder-width apart and slightly bend your knees. Take a step diagonally across your body with one foot, crossing it over the other leg, and then quickly push off with the crossed-over foot to propel yourself in the new direction. As you execute the crossover step, maintain a low and balanced stance to ensure stability and quick transitions.

This footwork technique is commonly used when moving laterally towards the Non-Volley Zone or when transitioning from baseline to net play. It allows you to cover ground rapidly and position yourself optimally for shots near the net. The crossover step is an essential footwork technique that enhances your court coverage and agility.

Cross step:

The **cross step** is a footwork technique that involves stepping across your body to change direction smoothly and swiftly. To execute the cross step correctly, start with your feet shoulder-width apart and slightly bend your knees. Take a step diagonally across your body with one foot, moving it towards the opposite side, and then quickly push off with the other foot to continue the movement.

As you perform the cross step, maintain a low and balanced stance to facilitate quick movements and ensure stability.

The cross step is particularly useful when transitioning from baseline to net play or when retrieving shots hit towards the corners of the court. It allows you to reposition yourself efficiently and maintain good court coverage, enabling you to respond effectively to a wide range of shots. The cross step enhances your agility and enables you to make seamless changes in direction on the pickleball court.

Mastering these footwork patterns will enhance your ability to reach shots effectively and maintain good court coverage.

Techniques for efficient movement and positioning on the court

Efficient movement and proper positioning on the court are essential for maintaining balance, reacting quickly, and executing shots effectively. Consider the following techniques:

- **Balanced stance**: Maintain a balanced stance with your feet shoulder-width apart, knees slightly bent, and weight evenly distributed on both feet. This stance provides a stable foundation for quick movements in any direction.
- **Step and slide**: When moving laterally, use small steps and slide your trailing foot to maintain balance and stability. This technique allows for quick changes in direction without losing control.
- **Small adjustment steps**: Make small adjustment steps to position yourself optimally for shots. These micro-movements allow you to set up for effective shot execution or quickly recover to defend against your opponent's shots.
- **Anticipate and prepare:** Anticipate your opponent's shots by reading their body language, racket (paddle) position, and court positioning. Position yourself strategically to be in an advantageous position for the next shot, whether it's an offensive attack or a defensive return.

By implementing these techniques, you will enhance your movement efficiency, court coverage, and overall performance on the pickleball court.

Strategies for anticipating and reacting to opponents' shots

Anticipating and reacting to your opponents' shots effectively can give you a competitive edge in pickleball. Consider these strategies:

- **Observe body language**: Pay attention to your opponent's body language, racket (paddle) preparation, and gaze to anticipate the direction and type of shot they are likely to play.
- **Visual focus**: Keep your eyes on the ball at all times, tracking its movement to react quickly and make accurate shot selections.
- **Stay alert and ready**: Maintain a high level of alertness and readiness, staying light on your feet and prepared to move in any direction.

- **Adjust positioning**: Continuously adjust your positioning on the court to maintain an advantageous position relative to your opponent's shot placement.
- **Develop court awareness**: Practice drills and play matches regularly to develop a keen sense of court awareness. This will enhance your ability to predict and react to your opponent's shots effectively.

By mastering footwork patterns, employing efficient movement techniques, and utilizing strategies for anticipating and reacting to opponents' shots, you will enhance your footwork skills, court coverage, and overall performance in pickleball. Regular practice and implementation of these techniques will help you become a more agile, precise, and successful player on the court.

CHAPTER 4   SERVING STRATEGIES

Welcome to **Chapter 4**, where we delve into the art of serving strategies in pickleball. Serving is a fundamental aspect of the game that sets the tone for each point and allows you to take control right from the start. In this chapter, we will unlock the secrets of effective serving, from mastering placement and spin to executing confident returns. Whether you're looking to improve your serving skills or enhance your ability to return your opponent's shots, this chapter will provide you with the techniques and insights you need to elevate your game to new heights. Get ready to unravel the mysteries of the serve and discover how to make a powerful impact on the court with your serves and returns.

4.1   SERVING SECRETS: PLACEMENT AND SPIN UNVEILED

The **serve** is a fundamental aspect of pickleball that sets the stage for each point. In this chapter, we will dive into the secrets of serving, focusing on techniques for achieving accurate and strategic serves, the importance of ball placement and targeting specific areas, and the effects of different types of spin on the serve. By mastering these elements, you can gain a significant advantage in your pickleball game.

It is important to note that the purpose of the serve (at the developing levels) is simply to place the ball in play and is not intended as an offensive weapon.

Techniques for achieving accurate and strategic serves

To enhance the accuracy and strategic nature of your serves, consider the following techniques:

- **Grip**: Maintain a firm but relaxed grip on the paddle, such as the continental grip or Eastern forehand grip. Experiment with different grips to find the one that provides you with optimal control and feel.
- **Stance and body positioning**: Adopt a balanced stance with your feet shoulder-width apart and your body aligned with the net. Position your non-dominant foot slightly ahead for stability and power generation.
- **Ball toss**: Develop a consistent and controlled ball toss by releasing the ball in front of you, slightly above eye level. Aim for a toss that allows you to make contact with the ball at the optimal height and position for your desired serve.
- **Racket (paddle) path**: Execute a smooth and fluid racket (paddle) path, starting from behind your body and moving upward to meet the ball at the highest point. This motion helps generate power, spin, and accuracy in your serve.
- **Follow-through**: Complete your serve with a full and controlled follow-through, extending your arm and racket (paddle) toward your target area. This follow-through helps maintain control and direction over the ball.

By incorporating these techniques into your serve, you can achieve greater accuracy, consistency, and strategic placement.

A **pre-serve routine** is a series of actions or rituals that a player goes through before serving the ball in pickleball. The specific actions can vary from player to player, but the goal is to establish a consistent routine that helps the player mentally and physically prepare for the serve.

Some examples of actions that might be included in a pre-serve routine include taking a deep breath, bouncing the ball a certain number of times, visualizing the serve, or adjusting the grip on the paddle. The key is to find a routine that works for you and helps you feel focused and confident before serving.

Having a pre-serve routine is recommended because it can help improve your serve by promoting consistency, focus, confidence, and relaxation. By going through the same routine before each serve, you can establish a consistent serving motion, block out distractions, and mentally prepare for the serve. This can help improve the accuracy and reliability of your serve and can also help you feel more confident and in control on the court.

Overall, a pre-serve routine is a valuable tool that can help you improve your serve and perform at your best in pickleball.

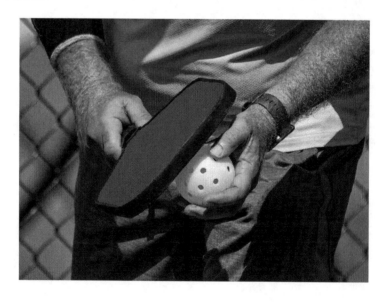

In pickleball, it is a rule that the server must announce the score before serving the ball. This ensures that all players are aware of the current score and helps prevent confusion or disputes. The server should clearly state the score, starting with their team's score followed by the opponent's score. In doubles pickleball, the server announces three numbers before serving the ball. The first number is the server's team score, the second number is the opponent's team score, and the third number indicates which server is serving (either 1 or 2).

For example, if the server's team has 3 points, the opponent's team has 5 points, and it is the first server's turn to serve, the server would say "3-5-1" before serving. Here is an example of what a player might say when announcing the score before serving in doubles pickleball:

Player: "The score is 3-5-1." (pauses to perform their pre-serve routine) "Ready?" (serves the ball)

However, it's important not to say the score and serve at the same time as it can distract from executing a proper serve. Announcing the score requires focus and attention, and trying to do it while serving can disrupt your serving routine and affect your accuracy and consistency. To avoid this, it is recommended to follow a specific sequence before serving the ball.

First, take a moment to think and mentally prepare for the serve. Then, clearly announce the score to ensure everyone is aware of the current score. After that, perform your pre-serve routine, such as bouncing the ball or adjusting your hat, to prepare yourself mentally and physically. Finally, execute your serve with focus and precision.

By following this sequence before each serve, you can improve your serving accuracy and consistency while maintaining clarity on the score. This helps create a fair and organized playing environment and enhances the overall experience of the game for all players.

Understanding the importance of ball placement and targeting specific areas

The serve in pickleball is the shot that starts the rally and gives you the opportunity to gain an advantage. It allows you to put the ball into play and dictate the pace of the game. A well-executed serve can give you the edge by putting pressure on your opponents and setting up favorable situations for your team. It is a crucial shot that can help you control the game and increase your chances of winning points.

Ball placement and targeting specific areas are crucial components of a successful serve. Consider the following aspects:

- **Targeting areas**: Analyze your opponent's positioning, weaknesses, and court coverage tendencies. Aim to serve to areas that exploit their vulnerabilities or force them out of their comfort zone. Targeting specific areas can vary, including deep corners, short angles, or even the body of your opponent.
- **Variation in placement**: Incorporate variation in your serves by targeting different areas of the court. Mix up serves to the forehand and backhand side, deep and short zones, or wide corners to keep your opponent guessing and off balance.
- **Court awareness**: Develop a keen sense of court awareness to read your opponent's positioning and adjust your serve placement accordingly. Observe their court coverage tendencies and adapt your serves to exploit gaps and weaknesses in their defense.

As a beginner, focus on serving to your opponent's weaker side or away from their dominant hand.

There are two serving techniques that are also useful to know:

Deep serve:

A **deep serve** in pickleball refers to a strategic serve that lands closer to the back boundary line of the receiving side. To execute a deep serve, focus on hitting the ball with more power and a higher trajectory. Aim for the back of the court, close to the baseline, to make it difficult for your opponent to return the ball effectively. The deep serve aims to force your opponent to move back and give you an advantage in the rally. It can create distance between the serving team and the receiving team, allowing the serving team to gain control of the point and potentially set up a favorable position for the next shot.

Short serve:

A **short serve** in pickleball is a serve that lands closer to the Non-Volley Zone or kitchen line on the receiving side. It is the opposite of the deep serve. It aims to land the ball just over the net, close to the Non-Volley Zone (kitchen). To execute a short serve, decrease your swing power and aim for a lower trajectory, ensuring the ball clears the net without bouncing too high. It is intentionally hit with less power and height, causing the ball to drop quickly and stay low over the net. This serve is designed to catch your opponent off guard and prevent them from making a strong return. The objective is to restrict the opponent's ability to attack and create opportunities for the serving team to move forward and take control of the net. By forcing the opponent to hit the ball from a less advantageous position, a short serve can disrupt their rhythm and limit their options for an aggressive return.

By strategically placing your serves and targeting specific areas, you can gain a tactical advantage and put pressure on your opponents.

Exploring different types of spin (topspin, backspin, sidespin) and their effects on the serve

Spin refers to the rotational movement imparted on the ball when it is struck. It alters the ball's trajectory, speed, and bounce, making it an invaluable tool for manipulating the game in your favor. By strategically applying spin to your serves, you can exploit your opponent's weaknesses, disrupt their rhythm, and gain a competitive edge.

Topspin:

Topspin is a type of spin where the ball rotates forward as it travels over the net. To execute a topspin serve, position the ball slightly closer to your non-dominant foot, and as you make contact with the ball, brush the paddle upwards and towards the ball with an accelerated motion. This action imparts a strong topspin on the ball, causing it to dip quickly after crossing the net. The topspin effect is created by the interaction between the paddle face and the ball's rotation.

Topspin serves are commonly employed to generate greater ball speed, increase accuracy, and enhance control. The pronounced downward trajectory created by topspin serves makes it challenging for your opponent to effectively handle the ball and execute a strong return.

Backspin:

Backspin, also known as underspin, involves rotating the ball backward as it moves towards your opponent. To execute a backspin serve, position the ball slightly closer to your dominant foot, and as you make contact with the ball, brush the paddle downwards and underneath the ball with a firm and controlled motion. This imparts a significant backspin on the ball, causing it to bounce lower and slower. The backspin effect creates a unique ball flight characterized by a lower bounce and reduced forward momentum.

Backspin serves are strategically used to disrupt your opponent's timing and rhythm, forcing them into defensive shots and limiting their ability to generate power in their return. The reduced bounce and slower pace of the ball make it more challenging for your opponent to execute aggressive shots, granting you greater control over the rally.

Sidespin:

Sidespin, also referred to as sideslice or cut, involves making the ball spin laterally, resulting in a curved trajectory. To execute a sidespin serve, position the ball slightly closer to the side of your dominant hand, and as you make contact with the ball, brush the paddle sideways across the ball with a deliberate and sweeping motion. This imparts a strong sidespin on the ball, causing it to deviate from its initial path and curve in the air.

Sidespin serves introduce an element of unpredictability and deception, as the ball veers off its expected trajectory after bouncing. This makes it challenging for your opponent to anticipate the ball's path and adjust their positioning and stroke accordingly. Sidespin serves can be particularly effective in creating confusion, disrupting your opponent's timing, and opening up opportunities for strategic shot placements.

Fast facts:

What are the rules for using **spin** when serving in pickleball?

According to the updated rules in 2023, the previously allowed one-handed pre-spun serve in pickleball is no longer permitted. This means players can't spin the ball using only one hand before serving. The updated USA Pickleball Rule Book will forbid applying any spin or manipulation of the ball from one hand, prior to striking it with the paddle for the serve.

To spin serve in pickleball, a player must use the non-paddle hand to toss the ball and the paddle hand to hit it perpendicular to the body. The non-paddle hand may impart spin on the ball, but the paddle or paddle hand may not2. The serve must be done with both feet behind the court's line and without letting the ball bounce.

By mastering these spin techniques and understanding when to utilize each type of serve, you can gain a significant advantage on the pickleball court. Experiment with different spin variations, placements, and speeds to further refine your serves and keep your opponents off balance. Developing a diverse and effective serving repertoire will not only enhance your ability to score points but also create opportunities to control the pace and dictate the flow of the game.

Fast facts:

An **ace** in pickleball occurs when the server hits the ball into the receiver's box, and the receiver fails to return the serve. It guarantees an immediate point and allows the server to move on to the next serve in the opposite box. Aces are not common in pickleball, but they provide a confident start to the next point. However, it is essential to prioritize consistent and inbounds serves to maintain control and maximize scoring opportunities. While aces are exciting, focusing on accuracy and minimizing errors ensures better chances of setting up favorable situations for winning points.

What are some **common mistakes beginners make** about **serving** and what are some **tips to remedy** them?

Grip inconsistency: One common mistake is having an inconsistent grip on the paddle during the serve. **Remedy**: Practice and find a grip that feels comfortable and secure.

Inconsistent toss: One common mistake is having an inconsistent toss, which can lead to inconsistent serves. **Remedy**: Practice and develop a consistent toss by focusing on a specific spot or target and using a gentle and controlled release of the ball. This helps in achieving a more accurate and reliable toss for a consistent serve.

Tossing the ball too low or too high: Beginners may struggle with tossing the ball at the appropriate height, leading to serving errors. **Remedy**: Practice and develop a consistent toss by aiming for a comfortable height that allows for better control over the serve.

Lack of proper paddle contact: Beginners may struggle with making solid paddle contact with the ball during the serve, resulting in weak or inconsistent serves. **Remedy**: Ensure proper paddle contact by aiming to strike the ball in the sweet spot of the paddle, which is typically near the center. This generates more power and control, leading to better serves.

Lack of proper weight transfer: Another common mistake is not transferring weight effectively during the serve, resulting in a weak or inaccurate shot. **Remedy**: Focus on shifting your weight from the back foot to the front foot during the serve, generating power and momentum.

Neglecting the follow-through: Beginners may sometimes neglect the follow-through after making contact with the ball, impacting the power and accuracy of the serve. **Remedy**: Ensure a complete follow-through by extending your arm and paddle towards the target.

Overhitting or underhitting the serve: These can result in the ball going out of bounds or falling short of the intended target. **Remedy**: Find the right balance by focusing on a controlled and smooth swing, using proper technique, and adjusting the power and angle of the paddle to achieve the desired placement and distance.

Lack of variety in serves: Beginners may often rely on one type of serve, limiting their options and making it easier for opponents to anticipate their shots. **Remedy**: Practice and develop different types of serves, such as the drive serve, lob serve, or drop serve. This adds variety to your game and keeps your opponents guessing.

Ignoring the service box boundaries: Beginners may unintentionally serve outside the designated service box boundaries, resulting in faults. **Remedy**: Pay close attention to the service box lines and ensure that the serve lands within the proper boundaries. Practice your aim and focus on hitting accurate serves to stay within the lines.

The following are examples of **drills** that a **beginner** could use to develop their skills in **serving**.

- **Target practice**: Set up targets on the opposite side of the court, such as hula hoops or cones, and aim to serve the ball into the targets. Start with larger targets and gradually decrease the size as you become more accurate.
- **Service line practice**: Stand at the baseline and focus on serving the ball over the net and landing it in the opponent's service box. Start with a slower and controlled serve, gradually increasing the speed and power as you progress.
- **Service box accuracy**: Choose a specific target within the opponent's service box, such as the corners or sidelines, and aim to consistently hit the target with your serves. This drill helps improve your ability to place the serve precisely.
- **Serve and run**: Serve the ball and quickly move towards the net to practice transitioning from the serve to the next shot. This drill helps improve your court positioning and readiness for the next shot after the serve.
- **Serve variation**: Practice different types of serves, such as the lob serve, drive serve, or spin serve. Experiment with different techniques and spins to develop a well-rounded serving game.
- **Serve and return**: Pair up with a practice partner and take turns serving and returning each other's serves. This drill helps simulate real game situations and improves your ability to respond to different types of serves.

Remember to focus on proper technique, such as a consistent toss and a smooth arm swing, during these drills. Start with slower serves and gradually increase the speed and complexity as you gain more confidence. Regularly practicing these serving drills will help you develop a reliable and effective serve in pickleball.

4.2   RETURN OF THE BALL: TECHNIQUES FOR CONFIDENT RETURNS

The **return of serve** refers to the shot played by the receiving player or team in response to the opponent's serve. It is the first stroke executed after the serve and marks the beginning of a rally. The return of serve is a crucial aspect of pickleball that can make or break a rally.

The primary objective of the return of serve is to effectively get the ball back into play, ideally with enough control and placement to disrupt the server's strategy and gain an advantageous position in the rally. The return of serve plays a crucial role in setting the tone for the rest of the point, as a well-executed return can put pressure on the server and provide an opportunity to gain an offensive advantage. Successful returns of serve often involve a combination of good footwork, anticipation, and shot placement to counteract the server's tactics and initiate a competitive rally.

In this section, we will explore techniques and strategies for confident returns, focusing on consistency, precision, footwork, positioning, and handling different types of serves. By mastering these skills, you can effectively neutralize your opponent's serve and gain control of the point.

Strategies for returning serves with consistency and precision

Consistency and precision are crucial elements in effectively returning serves in pickleball.

The first step in returning a serve is to position yourself correctly. Stand slightly behind the baseline and be prepared to move quickly. Keep your knees bent, weight on the balls of your feet, and your paddle up and ready. Anticipate the direction of the serve by watching your opponent's body language and racket (paddle) position.

When returning a serve, aim for consistency over power. Focus on getting the ball over the net and in play, rather than trying to hit a winner. Use a short, controlled swing to make contact with the ball and try to return it deep into your opponent's court. This will give you more time to recover and set up for the next shot.

It is important to stay mentally focused and maintain good court awareness when returning a serve. Pay attention to your opponent's positioning and be ready to adjust your shot based on their movement. Stay calm under pressure and avoid rushing your return.

To enhance your return game, it is important to implement the following strategies with meticulous attention to detail:

- **Focus and anticipation**: One of the first steps to returning serves with consistency and precision is to maintain a high level of focus. By carefully observing your opponent's stance, ball toss, and racket (paddle) angle, you can anticipate the trajectory and speed of the serve. This heightened awareness allows you to react swiftly and position yourself optimally to execute a solid return.
- **Controlled swing**: When returning a serve, it is essential to execute a controlled swing. This involves maintaining a compact and controlled backswing, which allows for precise contact with the ball. It is crucial to avoid overly aggressive swings that can lead to errors and inconsistent returns. By focusing on a controlled swing, you can ensure greater accuracy and increase your chances of a successful return.
- **Placement over power**: While power can be an asset, prioritizing ball placement over sheer force is often more effective when returning serves. Instead of solely relying on hitting the ball with maximum power, aim to direct the ball strategically into the opponent's court. Focus on placing the ball deep into their court or targeting specific areas that exploit their weaknesses or force them into challenging shot selections. This approach can give you an advantage by putting pressure on your opponent and creating opportunities for follow-up shots.
- **Watch the ball**: Throughout the entire process of returning a serve, it is crucial to maintain visual contact with the ball. From the moment the ball leaves your opponent's paddle until the point of contact, keep your eyes fixed on the ball. This unwavering focus ensures accurate timing and precise contact, enabling you to effectively control the return shot.

Play within a 'smaller court'. Avoid aiming for the opponent's baseline and instead target a few feet inside the baseline and sidelines. This approach will help minimize errors and prevent the pickleball from going out of bounds unnecessarily.

There are two techniques that are also useful to know:

One effective technique for returning a serve is the **soft drop shot**. This involves hitting the ball with a gentle touch, causing it to land close to the net and bounce low, making it difficult for your opponent to return. The soft drop shot is particularly effective against hard-hitting serves, as it takes away the power and forces your opponent to react quickly.

Another technique to consider is the **lob**. This shot is used when your opponent's serve is short and you have enough time to execute a high, arcing shot that clears the net and lands deep in your opponent's court. The lob can be a great way to disrupt your opponent's rhythm and force them to move quickly to retrieve the ball.

By diligently implementing these strategies, you can significantly improve your return consistency and strategically place the ball to gain an advantage over your opponent.

Fast facts:

What is the **Nasty Nelson**? The term "Nasty Nelson" in pickleball refers to a controversial strategy where a player intentionally hits the ball at an opponent's body, specifically targeting their upper body or head. This shot is aimed to create discomfort or intimidate the opponent, potentially causing them to make an error or lose their composure.

The Nasty Nelson is controversial because it goes against the principles of sportsmanship and fair play in pickleball. The sport is known for its friendly and inclusive nature, promoting good sportsmanship and respectful competition. Intentionally targeting an opponent with a hard-hit shot can be seen as unsportsmanlike behavior and may lead to injury or create a hostile environment on the court.

While pickleball encourages competitive play, players are expected to prioritize safety and respect for their opponents. The Nasty Nelson violates these principles and is generally discouraged in the pickleball community. It is important for players to maintain a positive and respectful approach to the game, focusing on skill, strategy, and fair play rather than resorting to aggressive or potentially dangerous tactics.

Footwork and positioning for optimal return placement

Footwork and positioning play a crucial role in setting up successful returns. Consider the following techniques:

- **Split-step**: Perform a split-step just as your opponent makes contact with the ball. This prepares your body for quick movement in any direction and allows for efficient weight transfer during the return.
- **Balanced stance:** Adopt a balanced stance with your feet shoulder-width apart and your body slightly forward. This enables quick lateral movement and stability during the return.
- **Adjusting position**: Anticipate the direction and trajectory of the serve to adjust your position accordingly. Move laterally or step forward to meet the ball at the ideal contact point for your desired return.

By mastering footwork and positioning, you can position yourself optimally for returns, allowing for greater control and placement.

Tips for handling different types of serves (hard, soft, spin)

Handling different types of serves in pickleball requires adaptability and a keen understanding of the serve's characteristics. To confidently return serves of varying types, consider the following detailed tips:

Hard serves:
When facing hard serves, maintaining focus is crucial. Adjust your timing to account for the increased speed of the ball. Use a shorter backswing to minimize the time it takes to prepare for the return. By meeting the ball slightly earlier, you can generate power and control. This adjustment allows you to effectively redirect the energy of the serve while maintaining accuracy.

Soft serves:
When dealing with soft serves, it's important to shift your approach to emphasize touch and finesse. Utilize a longer and controlled swing to match the slower pace of the serve. Instead of relying on power, focus on ball placement and precision. Direct the ball strategically to exploit openings in your opponent's court or force them into difficult shot selections. By emphasizing placement over power, you can maintain control and put your opponent on the defensive.

Spin serves:
Spin serves introduce a unique challenge due to the spin imparted on the ball. To handle spin serves effectively, anticipate the type and direction of the spin. This can be determined by observing your opponent's racket (paddle) angle and ball toss. Adjust your racket (paddle) angle and swing path accordingly to counteract the spin. For example, if the serve has topspin, position your racket (paddle) slightly below the ball's contact point and swing upward to neutralize the spin. By brushing against the spin, you can gain better control over the return and prevent the ball from veering off in unexpected directions.

By understanding and adapting to the different types of serves in pickleball, you can effectively handle various situations and maintain control during the return. Incorporating these detailed techniques into your game will enhance your consistency, precision, and overall ability to handle different serve types. As a result, you will gain a competitive edge and increase your chances of success in pickleball.

Top tips:

Anticipating the type of serve your opponent is about to make in pickleball can be challenging, but there are some tips that can help you:

- **Observe your opponent's pre-serve routine**: Pay attention to your opponent's pre-serve routine and body language. This can give you clues about the type of serve they are about to make.
- **Watch for changes in their serving pattern**: If your opponent has been consistently serving deep, for example, and suddenly changes to a short, angled serve, be prepared for this change and adjust your position accordingly.
- **Be ready for different types of serves**: Be aware of the different types of serves in pickleball, such as the power serve, **moon ball serve**, and short, angled serve. Be prepared to react to each type of serve and adjust your position accordingly.

By following these tips, you can improve your ability to anticipate the type of serve your opponent is about to make and react accordingly.

CHAPTER 5   THIRD SHOT TACTICS

Mastering the third shot is crucial in pickleball. In this **chapter**, we explore the techniques and strategies to excel in this important shot. From improving placement to creating opportunities and disrupting opponents, learn how to elevate your third shot game and enhance your overall strategy on the court.

Each point in pickleball follows a particular sequence: A player serves the pickleball for the first shot; an opponent returns the serve for the second shot; and the serving team either drives the pickleball or drops the pickleball for the third shot.

The **third shot** in pickleball is a pivotal element in the flow and outcome of a match. It's called the third shot because, following the serve (first shot) and the return of serve (second shot), it is the third hit of the ball in the rally.

In pickleball, the serving team is initially at a disadvantage because they must let the return of serve bounce once before hitting it, due to the double-bounce rule. This means that they have to execute their third shot while standing at the baseline, which can make it more difficult to regain control of the game.

The third shot is the serving team's first chance to regain control of the game and move forward from the baseline towards the net. Gaining control of the net, or the "kitchen" area (Non-Volley Zone), gives a team a significant advantage in pickleball. It allows for more aggressive volleying and limits the opposing team's options.

There are several options for a third shot, but the two most common ones are a **drive** and a **drop shot**.

A **drive** is a hard, low shot that can force the receiving team back, while a **drop shot** is soft and lands in the kitchen, making it difficult for the opposing team to attack. The choice between a drive and a drop shot as the third shot usually depends on the player's skills, the opponents' positioning, and the game's tempo.

Hence, the third shot is a critical tactical play in pickleball. Its importance lies in its potential to shift the game's dynamics, setting the stage for the serving team to take a more aggressive stance and seize control of the match. Mastering the third shot is often a key differentiator between novice and advanced pickleball players.

5.1   DRIVE TO SUCCEED: MASTERING THIRD SHOT DRIVES

Techniques for executing powerful and strategic third shot drives

Both power and strategy are important in the execution of the third shot drive in pickleball.

Power refers to the ability to generate sufficient force and speed in your shot. A powerful third shot drive allows you to hit the ball with enough velocity to clear the net and push your opponents back, putting them on the defensive. This power can be achieved through proper body positioning, generating momentum, and using an effective swing technique.

Strategic execution of the third shot drive involves considering the placement and direction of your shot. Instead of simply hitting the ball hard, a strategic approach focuses on targeting specific areas of the court that exploit weaknesses in your opponents' positioning or create difficulties in their shot selection. By strategically placing your third shot drive, you can gain an advantage and set yourself up for success in the rally.

When it comes to executing powerful and strategically effective third shot drives in pickleball, the following expanded tips can help enhance your game:

Grip:
Utilize a continental grip, where the paddle handle is held diagonally across the palm. This grip offers versatility in shot selection and enables you to generate both power and accuracy. By allowing a range of motion and flexibility in your wrist, the continental grip empowers you to adapt your shot to different situations, whether you need to add power or finesse to your drive.

Body positioning:
Maintain a balanced stance with a slight bend in the knees. This stance provides stability and creates a solid foundation for generating power in your shot. By keeping your body relaxed and your shoulders squared, you can effectively transfer energy from your core to your paddle. Face the direction of your intended target to align your body and focus your shot, enabling better control and accuracy.

Weight transfer:
As you approach the ball, shift your weight forward, transferring your body weight onto your front foot. This forward weight transfer is crucial for generating power and an aggressive shot. By channeling your momentum into the shot, you can add significant force to your third shot drive. Additionally, the weight transfer helps maintain balance and stability throughout your swing.

Timing:
Pay close attention to the timing of your swing, aiming to make contact with the ball at the optimal moment. Anticipate the ball's trajectory and adjust your timing accordingly. By synchronizing your swing with the incoming ball, you can maximize the power and control of your shot. Timing is particularly important for generating the desired power and precision required for a successful third shot drive.

Follow-through:
Complete your swing with a full and extended follow-through. The follow-through should be directed towards your intended target. This action not only enhances the power of your shot but also improves accuracy and control. A

proper follow-through allows you to guide the ball precisely to the desired location on the court, ensuring strategic placement and making it more challenging for your opponents to return the shot.

Understanding the role of placement, speed, and spin in effective drives

In pickleball, executing powerful drives is not only about hitting the ball with force but also understanding the importance of placement, speed, and spin. By strategically utilizing these elements, you can maximize the effectiveness of your drives and gain a competitive advantage over your opponents. In this section, we will delve into the significance of placement, speed, and spin in driving shots, providing you with the knowledge to make strategic decisions and elevate your game.

Placement:
Target specific areas of the court strategically to exploit weaknesses or create difficult angles, forcing your opponents into defensive positions. By aiming for the sidelines, corners, or open spaces, you can put pressure on your opponents and make it challenging for them to return your shots effectively. Thoughtful placement can disrupt your opponents' rhythm and give you opportunities to control the pace of the game.

Speed:
Varying the speed of your third shot drives is crucial in keeping your opponents off balance and preventing them from anticipating your shots. Mixing up the speed of your drives can create uncertainty for your opponents, making it difficult for them to adjust and respond effectively. By incorporating both fast-paced drives and slower, controlled shots, you can disrupt your opponents' timing and force errors.

Spin:
Spin is a powerful tool that can greatly influence the trajectory and behavior of the ball. By incorporating different types of spin into your drives, you can add an extra layer of complexity to your shots. Topsin, for example, can create a downward trajectory and increased bounce, making it challenging for your opponents to handle the ball. Backspin, on the other hand, provides more control and decreases the bounce, allowing for precise placement and drop shots. Sidespin can be utilized to change the direction of the ball, keeping your opponents guessing and making it harder for them to anticipate the path of your drives.

Understanding the role of placement, speed, and spin in effective drives gives you the ability to strategically manipulate the game and gain an upper hand. By incorporating these elements into your drives, you can control the tempo, create opportunities for winners, and keep your opponents on their toes. Experiment with different placement strategies, vary your shot speeds, and explore the potential of spin to enhance your drives and take your game to the next level.

Tips for varying shot selection based on court positioning and opponents' positioning

Here are some tips for varying shot selection based on court positioning and opponents' positioning:

- **Assess court positioning**: Pay attention to your position on the court and the position of your opponents. Adjust your shot selection based on whether you are near the net, in the middle of the court, or at the baseline. Take note of your opponents' positions as well, as it can influence the effectiveness of certain shots.
- **Use drop shots**: When your opponents are positioned farther back on the court, consider using drop shots to force them to move forward and make it difficult for them to return the ball effectively. Drop shots can catch your opponents off guard and create opportunities for you to gain control of the point.
- **Employ lobs**: If your opponents are positioned close to the net or if they have a weak overhead shot, utilizing lobs can be an effective strategy. Lobs allow you to hit the ball high and deep, forcing your opponents to move back and giving you time to regain a favorable position on the court.
- **Aim for the sidelines**: When your opponents are out of position or have limited court coverage, targeting the sidelines can be a smart choice. By hitting wide shots, you can exploit the open space and make it difficult for your opponents to reach the ball in time, increasing the likelihood of scoring a point.
- **Adjust shot pace**: Varying the pace of your shots can disrupt your opponents' rhythm and make it challenging for them to anticipate your next move. Mix up the speed of your shots by alternating between fast drives and slower, controlled shots. This unpredictability can create confusion and give you the upper hand in rallies.
- **Utilize angles:** Look for opportunities to hit angled shots that force your opponents to cover a larger distance on the court. By directing the ball away from the center and towards the corners, you can create wider angles that require your opponents to stretch and potentially open up the court for your next shot.
- **Exploit weaknesses**: Observe your opponents' strengths and weaknesses and adjust your shot selection accordingly. If they struggle with backhand shots, for example, target that side of the court more frequently. Exploiting weaknesses can put your opponents under pressure and give you an advantage in the match.
- **Stay adaptable**: Be flexible in your shot selection and adapt to the changing dynamics of the game. As the match progresses, the court positioning and opponents' tactics may evolve. Stay observant and adjust your shot selection to maintain a competitive edge.

By varying your shot selection based on court positioning and opponents' positioning, you can keep your opponents guessing, exploit their vulnerabilities, and control the flow of the game. Assess the situation, use a combination of drop shots, lobs, angled shots, and targeted placements to keep your opponents off balance and maximize your chances of success on the pickleball court.

5.2 DROP SHOT DELIGHTS: PERFECTING THIRD SHOT DROPS

Exploring the art of executing controlled and deceptive third shot drops

The ability to execute precise and deceptive third shot drops is crucial in pickleball as it allows you to regain control of the point, put pressure on your opponents, and create opportunities for offensive plays. In this section, we will delve into the techniques and strategies for mastering the art of executing controlled and deceptive third shot drops.

- **Soft touch**: Develop a delicate touch and control over the ball to execute precise and gentle third shot drops. Use minimal force and rely on finesse to softly land the ball near the kitchen line.
- **Feathering the shot**: Master the technique of "feathering" the shot, which involves reducing the impact of the paddle on the ball to create a slow and controlled descent. This technique adds unpredictability and makes it challenging for opponents to anticipate the trajectory of the ball.
- **Angle selection**: Choose the appropriate angle for your third shot drops based on the court positioning of your opponents. Aim for angles that force your opponents to cover more distance or retrieve the ball from difficult positions.
- **Placement near the kitchen line**: Focus on placing the third shot drop close to the kitchen line to limit your opponents' options and put pressure on them to execute a precise and controlled response.

Understanding the importance of touch, finesse, and angle selection

Touch, finesse, and angle selection are key elements in executing effective and strategic third shot drops in pickleball. They involve specific skills and techniques that contribute to the success of your shots. Let's explore what each term means and how they contribute to your overall game.

Touch:
Touch refers to the delicate control and feel you have over the ball during your shots. It involves the ability to make subtle adjustments in your grip, paddle contact, and the amount of force applied to the ball. Developing good touch allows you to manipulate the ball's trajectory and placement with precision.

Finesse:
Finesse is the art of executing shots with finesse involves using soft hands and a gentle touch to generate just enough power to clear the net and land the ball in the desired location. It is about finesse, accuracy, and control rather than relying solely on power. Finesse shots require a delicate balance between power and touch, allowing you to place the ball with precision.

Angle selection:

Angle selection refers to the strategic use of angles in your shots. It involves hitting the ball in a way that creates difficult-to-reach shots for your opponents. By choosing the right angle, you can force your opponents to cover more distance or take shots from unfavorable positions. Angle selection adds an element of strategy and complexity to your game.

Tips for executing controlled and deceptive third shot drops:

✓ Develop soft hands and a light grip to enhance your touch and control over the ball.
✓ Focus on placing your drop shots close to the net and near the sidelines to create difficult angles for your opponents.
✓ Vary the pace and spin of your drop shots to keep your opponents off balance.
✓ Experiment with different angles when executing third shot drops to catch your opponents off guard.
✓ Use subtle body and paddle movements to deceive your opponents and maintain the element of surprise.
✓ Practice drills that specifically target touch and control to improve your finesse.
✓ Observe your opponents' positioning and movement patterns to identify their weaknesses and exploit them with well-placed drop shots.
✓ Stay balanced and ready, maintaining a balanced stance and being prepared to quickly transition from your previous shot.
✓ Continuously evaluate the effectiveness of your drop shots and make adjustments to your technique and strategy.
✓ Develop a feel for the game by practicing regularly and gaining experience in executing third shot drops with precision.

By mastering touch, finesse, and angle selection, you will be able to execute controlled and deceptive third shot drops that can give you an advantage in your pickleball game.

Strategies for placing drops in difficult-to-reach areas for opponents

Placing third shot drops in difficult-to-reach areas is a strategic advantage in pickleball. By targeting specific areas of the court, you can force your opponents into awkward positions and limit their shot options. In this section, we will discuss various strategies and techniques for placing drops in challenging locations, giving you an upper hand in dictating the flow of the game.

- **Observe court coverage of opponents**: Pay attention to your opponents' movement and court coverage patterns. Identify areas of the court that they may struggle to reach quickly or anticipate well.
- **Utilize sideline and corner placements**: Aim for the sidelines and corners of the court to place the third shot drop in areas that require your opponents to cover a larger distance. This increases the likelihood of forcing them into errors or weak returns.

- **Vary drop placement**: Mix up your drop shot placements to keep your opponents off balance. Alternate between cross-court drops, deep sideline drops, and short angle drops to create unpredictability and make it difficult for your opponents to anticipate your shots.
- **Use deceptive shots**: Incorporate deceptive shots by disguising your intention to hit a drop shot. Initially, use a similar setup and body positioning as when executing other shots to confuse your opponents and make it harder for them to read your drop shots.

Top tips:

Shake 'N' Bake is a term used to describe a play in doubles pickleball where the serving team follows up the serve with an aggressive and quick volley or shot, putting pressure on the opponent and aiming to win the point. This strategy is popular amongst aggressive-style pickleball players and can be extremely effective if executed properly.

In a Shake 'N' Bake play, one partner of the serving team drives the third shot, while the other partner crashes (i.e., runs to) the pickleball net. The third shot is a key component of this strategy, as it sets up the opportunity for the partner at the net to put away the fifth shot if the opposing team pops the drive up into the air. The partner that crashes or runs to the pickleball net is trying to put away the fifth shot. This strategy relies on effective communication and individual skill of the teammates.

The success of a Shake 'N' Bake play depends on several factors, including hitting a quality third shot that is low over the pickleball net, having strong placement of the third shot to attack the weaker of the two opposing players, and moving your feet quickly to crash the pickleball net. If executed properly, a Shake 'N' Bake play can put a ton of pressure on opposing pickleball players and help you gain control of the rally and win points.

By mastering the art of executing controlled and deceptive third shot drops, understanding the importance of touch, finesse, and angle selection, and implementing strategies to place drops in difficult-to-reach areas, you can enhance your overall game and gain an advantage over your opponents in pickleball. These techniques will enable you to execute precise and effective third shot drops that keep your opponents on their toes and create opportunities for you to take control of the point.

CHAPTER 6   CRAFTY TACTICS

In **Chapter 6**, we dive into the exciting world of offensive and defensive tactics in pickleball. This chapter is all about unleashing your skills to create a strong game that combines precision, power, and strategic thinking. **Offensive shots** allow you to seize control of the game, put your opponents on the defensive, and create opportunities to dominate rallies. On the other hand, **defensive strategies** help you react and respond effectively to your opponent's attacks, maintaining control and turning the tide of the game in your favor. We will explore a range of topics including shot selection, techniques for generating power and accuracy, as well as defensive strategies to anticipate and counter your opponent's moves.

6.1   RALLYING AND SHOT SELECTION

For a new pickleball player, understanding the art of rallying and shot selection is key to mastering the game.

Rallying is the heart of pickleball, where both teams exchange shots, aiming to keep the ball in play. It is crucial to develop consistency in your shots, which comes with practice and proper technique. Begin by focusing on your footwork and positioning. Ensure that you are always balanced and ready to move in any direction. This will allow you to react quickly and reach the ball effectively.

Shot selection is about making the right decision at the right time. It requires analyzing the situation, understanding your opponents' weaknesses, and exploiting them. One fundamental principle is to avoid unforced errors. Instead of going for risky shots, aim for consistent and controlled shots that keep the ball in play. This will put pressure on your opponents and increase your chances of winning the point.

6.2   OFFENSIVE WIZARDRY: CRAFTING SHOTS FOR PRECISION AND POWER

Offensive shots in pickleball refer to aggressive and attacking shots that are aimed at putting pressure on the opponent and winning points. These shots are designed to take control of the rally, dictate the pace, and force the opponent into defensive positions.

Offensive shots in pickleball include powerful **drives**, **smashes**, and well-placed **volleys** that are aimed to score points outright or set up an advantageous position for the next shot.

These shots are characterized by their speed, precision, and the intention to gain an advantage by placing the ball in areas that are difficult for the opponent to return effectively.

Offensive shots are crucial in maintaining an offensive strategy and keeping the opponent on the defensive, increasing the chances of winning the rally.

Exploring offensive shot selection and execution

Offensive shot selection and execution are crucial elements in unleashing your attacking prowess on the pickleball court. It involves choosing the right shots at the right time and executing them with precision and intent. Let's delve into the world of offensive shot selection and discover the shots that can help you gain the upper hand in your matches.

Drive shots:
Master the art of the drive shot, which involves hitting the ball forcefully and aggressively towards your opponent's side of the court. This shot aims to put your opponent under pressure, forcing them to defend and creating opportunities to attack.

Smash shots:
Unleash the power of the smash shot, a powerful overhead shot that aims to drive the ball downwards with immense force. The smash shot is often executed when the ball is high and provides an excellent opportunity to overwhelm your opponents with its speed and intensity.

Drop shots:
Employ the element of surprise with well-executed drop shots. These shots involve delicately guiding the ball over the net and landing it softly and close to the net on your opponent's side. Drop shots can catch your opponents off guard, forcing them to rush forward and potentially creating openings for more aggressive shots.

Techniques for generating power and accuracy in aggressive shots

Power and accuracy are the foundations of effective offensive shots. To craft shots that combine both power and precision, it is essential to master specific techniques that allow you to generate maximum force while maintaining control. Let's explore techniques that will help you unleash your offensive prowess.

- **Utilize proper weight transfer**: Shift your weight forward and use your entire body to generate power in your shots. Initiating the shot with your legs and transferring your body weight into the shot will add explosive power to your offensive shots.
- **Maintain a firm grip**: Ensure you have a secure grip on the paddle to maintain control and accuracy while generating power. A loose grip can result in loss of control and accuracy, compromising the effectiveness of your offensive shots.
- **Use rotational power**: Engage your core muscles and incorporate rotational power into your shots. Rotating your hips and shoulders in sync with your swing will allow you to generate additional power and torque, resulting in more forceful and impactful shots.

Strategies for creating opportunities to attack and dominate rallies

Crafting offensive shots is not just about individual techniques; it is also about creating opportunities to attack and dominate rallies. By implementing strategic tactics and reading the game effectively, you can set yourself up for offensive success. Let's explore some strategies for creating openings to attack.

- **Capitalize on weak returns**: Identify weak returns from your opponents and exploit them by aggressively attacking with powerful shots. Look for opportunities when your opponents' shots lack depth, pace, or accuracy, and use these openings to seize control of the rally.
- **Control the center of the court**: Aim to position yourself at the center of the court, which allows you to have better court coverage and provides the opportunity to attack from a more advantageous position. Dominating the center court position puts you in control of the rally and forces your opponents into defensive positions.
- **Utilize effective shot placement**: Strategically place your offensive shots to exploit openings or exploit your opponents' weaknesses. Target specific areas on the court, such as sidelines, corners, or the "no-volley zone," to create challenging situations for your opponents. Aim for spots where they have difficulty reaching or executing shots. Precise and consistent shot placement puts you in control and increases your chances of scoring.

Top tips:

An **approach shot** in pickleball is a shot that is hit while moving in a forward motion towards the pickleball net. It is typically an offensive shot, as it allows you to move closer to the net and take control of the point.

Here are some **tips** for executing an approach shot in pickleball:

- ✓ Look for opportunities to hit an approach shot when your opponent hits a weak or short shot.
- ✓ Aim to hit the ball deep into your opponent's court, forcing them to hit a defensive shot.
- ✓ Hit the ball with good pace and placement, making it difficult for your opponent to return the ball effectively.
- ✓ Move towards the net as you hit the approach shot, allowing you to get into a better position to control the point.

Top tips:

In pickleball, an "attack" refers to an aggressive shot or strategy aimed at gaining an advantage over the opponent. It involves hitting powerful or well-placed shots to put pressure on the opponent and create scoring opportunities. The goal is to control the point and force the opponent into a defensive position. Successful attacks require power, accuracy, and strategic shot selection to exploit the opponent's weaknesses.

6.3 DEFENSIVE STRATEGIES: NAVIGATING THE COURT WITH SMARTS

In this section, we dive into the realm of **defensive strategies**, where intelligence and positioning play a critical role in neutralizing your opponents' aggressive shots.

Defensive play requires a keen understanding of shot selection, precise positioning, and the ability to counter your opponents' attacking shots. By mastering the art of defense, you can frustrate your opponents' offensive efforts and maintain control of the game. Let's explore the key elements of defensive strategies and elevate your defensive game to new heights.

Understanding defensive shot selection and positioning

Defensive shot selection and positioning form the foundation of effective defensive play in pickleball. These shots are employed in response to an opponent's aggressive play, with the goal of maintaining control and prolonging the rally. They are characterized by strategic placement and trajectory, often aiming deep into the opponent's court or targeting challenging areas. Consistency, accuracy, and controlled power take precedence over aggressive shot placement in defensive play. Mastering these techniques will help you become a formidable defensive player in pickleball.

Common defensive shots in pickleball include:

Deep lobs:
These shots are hit high and deep into the opponent's court, aiming to push them back and buy time to recover or reposition defensively. Deep lobs force opponents to hit overhead shots, giving the defending player an opportunity to regain control of the rally.

Dinks:
Dinks are soft and controlled shots executed close to the net. They require precise touch and finesse, allowing players to slow down the pace of the game and create opportunities for strategic positioning. Dinks are effective in neutralizing aggressive shots from opponents and forcing them to play more defensively.

Block shots:
Block shots involve absorbing the pace and power of an opponent's shot by lightly redirecting the ball back over the net. This defensive shot requires good timing, as it aims to neutralize the opponent's aggression without generating significant power. Block shots are commonly used when defending against hard-hitting shots or smashes.

Cross-court shots:
When playing defensively, hitting shots cross-court can be advantageous. Cross-court shots allow players to create wider angles, forcing opponents to cover more ground and increasing the likelihood of their shot falling outside the opponent's comfortable hitting zone.

Techniques for effectively countering opponents' aggressive shots

Effectively countering your opponents' aggressive shots is a key component of defensive play. It requires a combination of skill, anticipation, and quick reflexes to neutralize your opponents' attacks and turn the tables in your favor. Let's explore techniques that will help you become a master at countering your opponents' aggressive shots.

- **Quick footwork**: Develop agile footwork to quickly react to your opponents' shots and position yourself optimally for a defensive response. Quick movements and adjustments will allow you to reach challenging shots and maintain your defensive stance.
- **Soft hands**: Cultivate soft hands to absorb the power of your opponents' shots and execute controlled and accurate returns. By maintaining a relaxed grip and allowing the paddle to absorb the ball's impact, you can return shots with precision and reduce the risk of errors.
- **Anticipation**: Sharpen your ability to anticipate your opponents' shots by reading their body language, racket (paddle) position, and shot patterns. Anticipating the direction and pace of incoming shots will enable you to react more quickly and effectively.

Importance of anticipation, court coverage, and controlled placement in defensive play

In defensive play, the elements of anticipation, court coverage, and controlled placement play crucial roles in neutralizing your opponents' attacks and gaining the upper hand. By understanding and applying these principles, you can become a formidable defender on the pickleball court.

Let's explore the meaning and significance of anticipation, court coverage, and controlled placement in defensive play.

Anticipation:
Anticipation in defensive play refers to the ability to read and predict your opponents' shots before they are executed. It involves observing their body language, footwork, and shot preparation to anticipate the direction, pace, and spin of the incoming shot. Anticipation allows you to position yourself strategically, react quickly, and prepare for an effective defensive response.

- ✓ Watch your opponent's body language and shot preparation to anticipate the direction of their shot.
- ✓ Pay attention to their court positioning and the angle of their racket (paddle) to gauge the potential shot placement.
- ✓ Anticipate the pace and spin of the incoming shot by observing the racket's (paddle's)contact point with the ball.
- ✓ Stay focused and mentally engaged throughout the point to react quickly to your opponent's shots.
- ✓ Practice reading your opponent's patterns and tendencies to improve your anticipation skills over time.

Court coverage:

Court coverage encompasses the movement and positioning on the court to ensure you can effectively reach and respond to your opponents' shots. It involves efficiently moving to cover all areas of the court, from side to side and forward to the net. Good court coverage allows you to maintain a strong defensive stance and retrieve challenging shots while minimizing gaps that your opponents can exploit.

✓ Maintain an athletic stance with knees slightly bent, allowing for quick movement in all directions.
✓ Utilize efficient footwork techniques, such as quick shuffles and split steps, to cover the court effectively.
✓ Anticipate the most likely areas your opponent will target and position yourself accordingly.
✓ Use lateral movements to cover the width of the court, and quick forward and backward movements to cover the depth.
✓ Develop good court awareness by constantly scanning the court and adjusting your positioning in response to your opponent's shots.

Controlled placement:

Controlled placement refers to the intentional and strategic placement of your defensive shots. It involves hitting the ball with precision and accuracy to specific areas of the court that make it difficult for your opponents to launch effective attacks. By placing your shots away from your opponents' preferred hitting zones or into areas that force them into defensive positions, you can disrupt their offensive rhythm and gain control of the rally.

✓ Aim for deep shots to push your opponent towards the back of the court, limiting their offensive options.
✓ Hit shots close to the sidelines to force your opponent to cover a larger area, increasing the likelihood of an error.
✓ Mix up the pace and trajectory of your shots to keep your opponent off balance and guessing.
✓ Target the weaker side of your opponent to exploit their vulnerabilities.
✓ Practice precision and consistency in your shots to ensure that you can place the ball exactly where you want it.

Now that we have explored the meaning and importance of anticipation, court coverage, and controlled placement, let's dive deeper into specific techniques and strategies to enhance your defensive skills and become a formidable force on the pickleball court.

6.4 DOUBLES CHEMISTRY: COMMUNICATION AND COORDINATION

Communication on the pickleball court is crucial for coordinating shots, anticipating opponents' moves, and ensuring efficient coverage of the court.

In doubles play, effective communication and coordination with your partner are essential for success on the pickleball court. It's not just about individual skills, but also about working together as a team to maximize your performance and outsmart your opponents.

This section will explore the importance of communication and coordination in doubles play and provide strategies for enhancing your doubles chemistry.

Importance of effective communication and teamwork in doubles play

In doubles pickleball, communication and teamwork are key factors that can significantly impact your performance on the court. This section explores the crucial role of effective communication and teamwork in maximizing your success as a doubles team. It starts with establishing clear signals and a common language with your partner.

✓ Establish clear and open lines of communication with your partner from the start of the match.
✓ Communicate your intentions, such as shot selection, court positioning, and strategies, to avoid confusion and overlap.
✓ Utilize verbal cues, hand signals, or predetermined signals to indicate shot intentions, positioning, and tactics. This will help you avoid confusion and make split-second decisions with ease.
✓ Maintain continuous communication throughout the match, providing feedback, encouragement, and support to your partner.
✓ Develop a sense of trust and understanding with your partner, which will allow for more effective coordination and decision-making on the court.

Regularly discuss your game plan, strengths, weaknesses, and adjustments needed during the match. Sharing feedback and offering support will help you both improve your skills and make necessary adjustments to outsmart your opponents.

Strategies for coordinating shot selection and court positioning with a partner

Coordinating shot selection and court positioning with your doubles partner is essential for a well-rounded and cohesive game plan.

This section delves into strategies and techniques that will help you synchronize your shot choices and court positioning to optimize your doubles performance.

✓ Understand each other's strengths, weaknesses, and preferred playing styles through regular practice and observation.
✓ Coordinate shot selection based on each player's strengths, taking advantage of their specific skills and abilities.
✓ Adapt your shot selection based on the specific situation in the match, such as adjusting the pace, angle, or placement of your shots.
✓ Work together to establish a balanced court coverage, ensuring that both players are positioned optimally to cover the court effectively.
✓ Maintain awareness of your partner's positioning and movements on the court to avoid collisions and maximize court coverage.

Tips for maximizing the strengths of each player and exploiting opponents' weaknesses

Understanding and leveraging the strengths of each player while capitalizing on your opponents' weaknesses can give you a competitive edge in doubles play.

This section provides valuable tips and insights on how to identify, enhance, and utilize your strengths as a team to outsmart and outplay your opponents.

✓ Identify and capitalize on your partner's strengths, whether it's their powerful serves, quick reflexes, or strategic shot placement.
✓ Communicate and adjust tactics to exploit your opponents' weaknesses, such as targeting their weaker side or exploiting gaps in their court coverage.
✓ Develop specific strategies and plays that play to your partner's strengths and put pressure on the opposing team.
✓ Take advantage of opportunities to create offensive plays, such as setting up your partner for a winning shot or executing effective poaching strategies.
✓ Adapt your game plan based on the strengths and weaknesses of your opponents, adjusting your shots and strategies accordingly.

By emphasizing effective communication, coordinating shot selection and court positioning, and maximizing each player's strengths, you can enhance your doubles chemistry and elevate your performance on the pickleball court. Remember, doubles play is not just about individual skills, but about the synergy and teamwork between you and your partner.

Top tips:

What is a **half stack**? In pickleball, the term "half stack" refers to a specific court positioning strategy employed by the serving team in doubles play. In a half stack formation, the serving team's players align themselves closer to the centerline, with one player positioned at the Non-Volley Zone (NVZ) line and the other player slightly behind and towards the middle of the court.

This formation allows the serving team to have better court coverage and strategic advantage during the serve. The player at the NVZ line is ready to engage in a quick and aggressive volley, while the player at the back provides additional court coverage and can handle deeper shots or defensive situations. The half stack formation enables the serving team to control the game's tempo, apply pressure on the opponents, and create opportunities for offensive plays. It is a popular strategy used by skilled doubles players to gain an advantage during the serve and maintain control of the rally.

Doubles – summing up some basic strategies for beginners

Playing doubles pickleball is a fantastic way to enjoy the sport while fostering teamwork and communication with your partner. As a beginner, understanding some fundamental strategies can greatly improve your performance on the court and enhance the overall experience. In this section, we'll cover the basic strategies for playing doubles pickleball.

Court positioning and movement:
✓ **Divide the court**: The court can be divided into three zones - forecourt, midcourt, and backcourt. At the beginning of each rally, position yourself strategically to cover different areas efficiently.
✓ **Stay side-by-side**: Maintain a side-by-side formation with your partner to minimize gaps in your defense and to communicate effectively during play.
✓ **Move as a unit**: Work as a team and move in sync with your partner. Avoid crowding one area and leave no openings for your opponents to exploit.

Serving strategies:
✓ **Get your serve in**: As a beginner, focus on consistency rather than power. Getting your serve in play is more important than trying to hit a powerful serve that might result in errors.
✓ **Aim for the deep court**: Place your serve deep into the opponent's court to force them to move back and create opportunities for your team to gain control of the net.

Return of serve:
✓ **Keep it low and controlled**: Aim for a soft and controlled return, preferably a dink, to avoid giving your opponents an easy opportunity to attack.
✓ **Direct returns away from the server**: Hit returns away from the server to make it difficult for them to follow up at the net.

Third-shot strategies:
✓ **Opt for a drop shot**: In most situations, play a drop shot for your third shot to keep the ball low and force your opponents to hit upward, limiting their attacking options.
✓ **Be ready for the net**: After hitting the third shot, quickly move to the net to assume an offensive position.

Dinking and the kitchen game:
✓ **Master the dink shot**: Dinking is a crucial skill in doubles pickleball. Work on developing soft and precise shots to keep your opponents out of their comfort zone.
✓ **Utilize the kitchen**: Stay close to the Non-Volley Zone (kitchen) to control the game and put pressure on your opponents.

Communication and signals:
✓ **Talk to your partner**: Maintain open communication with your partner throughout the match. Call out shots, provide encouragement, and discuss strategies.

✓ **Use non-verbal cues**: Develop non-verbal signals to coordinate movements and indicate your intentions during fast-paced rallies.

As a beginner playing doubles pickleball, the key is to focus on communication, court positioning, and consistency. Work together with your partner, support each other, and remember to have fun. By following these basic strategies and practicing regularly, you'll build a strong foundation for successful doubles play and enjoy the game even more. Keep learning, stay positive, and embrace the camaraderie that makes doubles pickleball such a delightful sport for players of all levels.

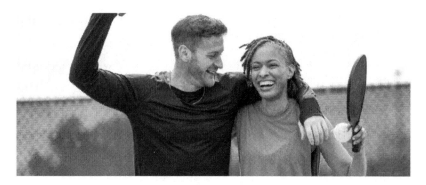

6.5   THE SINGLES GAME

One of the great things about pickleball is its versatility. Whether you prefer playing with a partner or flying solo, there's a game style that suits everyone's tastes. In this subchapter, we will explore the differences between doubles and singles play, giving new pickleball players a clearer understanding of both formats.

Doubles play is the most popular and widely played version of pickleball. It involves teams of two players on each side, with partners standing on opposite sides of the net. Doubles play allows for greater teamwork and strategic coordination between partners. It's a fantastic way to socialize and build camaraderie on the court. Playing doubles also means you have an additional person to cover more ground, increasing your chances of returning shots effectively.

On the other hand, **singles play** is a one-on-one game where each player occupies the entire court. This format requires players to be more physically fit and strategically agile since they have to cover the entire court themselves. Singles play often demands more stamina and quick reflexes, making it a great option for players who enjoy a more intense and challenging experience.

Choosing between doubles and singles play ultimately comes down to personal preference. If you enjoy teamwork and socializing, doubles play may be the perfect fit for you. It allows for continuous communication with your partner, strategizing together, and sharing the joy of victories. Doubles play is also an excellent opportunity to develop your skills, as you can observe and learn from your partner's techniques.

On the other hand, singles play offers a chance for individual growth and self-improvement. It allows you to focus solely on your own game, sharpening your skills and building stamina. Singles play can be a more physically demanding experience, but it can also provide a sense of accomplishment and personal achievement when you conquer the court alone.

As a beginner, it's highly recommended to start with doubles play. It provides a supportive environment where you can learn from your partner and understand the dynamics of the game more easily. Once you feel more confident and comfortable with the basics, you can explore the challenges of singles play.

Remember, whether you choose doubles or singles play, the most important thing is to enjoy the game and have fun. Pickleball is a sport that can be enjoyed at any skill level, and both formats offer unique experiences and opportunities for growth.

Some tips for playing singles

For new pickleball players, the game of singles pickleball is an exciting and challenging way to fully immerse yourself in this fast-paced sport. While doubles pickleball is often the preferred choice for beginners, singles play offers a unique experience that allows you to focus on your individual skills, strategy, and overall game improvement. In this subchapter, we will delve into the world of singles pickleball and provide you with essential tips and techniques to help you succeed on the court.

One of the key differences between singles and doubles pickleball is the increased amount of court coverage required in singles play. Without a partner to rely on, you must be prepared to cover the entire court and anticipate your opponent's shots. This means staying light on your feet, constantly adjusting your position, and being ready to move quickly in all directions. Developing good footwork and agility is crucial for success in singles pickleball.

Another important aspect of singles play is shot selection. With no partner to assist you, it's essential to choose your shots wisely and exploit your opponent's weaknesses. This requires a combination of power, accuracy, and finesse. Mastering a variety of shots, such as drives, drops, lobs, and dinks, will give you a competitive edge and allow you to control the pace of the game.

In singles pickleball, strategy is key. You must be able to read your opponent's movements, anticipate their shots, and adjust your own game plan accordingly. Understanding when to be aggressive and when to play defensively can make a significant difference in your performance. Additionally, learning to manage your energy and stamina throughout the match is crucial for maintaining a consistent level of play.

While singles pickleball may seem daunting at first, it offers tremendous opportunities for growth and improvement. Embrace the challenge, focus on developing your individual skills, and enjoy the thrill of competing one-on-one. As a beginner, it's important to remember that practice and patience are essential. With time and dedication, you'll become more confident in your abilities and find great satisfaction in your progress.

Fast facts:

Cutthroat pickleball is a variation of the game that involves three players instead of the traditional two. In this version, one player is designated as the "solo" player, while the other two players are on a team. The solo player must try to win points against both members of the opposing team. The solo player rotates after each point, giving everyone a chance to play offense and defense.

Singles – summing up some basic strategies for beginners

Because pickleball can be played in both singles and doubles formats, each requires different strategies. In singles pickleball, you'll be alone on one side of the court, which means you must adapt your approach to suit the unique challenges of the game.

In singles pickleball, the court coverage takes on a different dimension, as you find yourself alone on one side of the court. This means you have the sole responsibility of covering the entire court, necessitating quick and efficient movement to retrieve shots effectively. Unlike in doubles play, there are fewer interactions with a partner in singles, leading to limited communication opportunities. As a result, you must rely solely on your own decision-making throughout the match. Another crucial aspect of singles strategy is the constant need to alternate between offensive and defensive positions. This dynamic approach is necessary as you switch from attacking to defending rapidly, making every shot and movement critical in singles play.

This section will provide you with some basic strategies tailored to singles play.

Positioning and movement:
✓ **Stay balanced**: Maintain a balanced stance, ready to move in any direction quickly.
✓ **Center of the court**: Return to the center after each shot to cover more court area effectively.

Serving strategies:
✓ **Start strong**: Begin with a powerful and well-placed serve to gain an advantage in the rally.
✓ **Mix it up**: Alternate between different serves (drive, lob, slice) to keep your opponent guessing.

Return of serve:
- ✓ **Stay aggressive**: Take advantage of weak serves by returning aggressively and aiming to control the rally from the start.
- ✓ **Limit errors**: Focus on getting your return in play to avoid giving free points to your opponent.

Third-shot strategies:
- ✓ **Plan ahead**: Anticipate the opponent's shot after your serve and be ready to react.
- ✓ **Utilize drop shots**: Opt for drop shots to initiate dinking rallies and gain control of the net.

Dinking and the kitchen game:
- ✓ **Master the dink**: Develop precise dinking skills to maneuver your opponent and create opportunities for winners.
- ✓ **Mind the kitchen**: Stay close to the Non-Volley Zone (kitchen) and avoid volleying from the baseline.

Balance offense and defense:
- ✓ **Know when to attack**: Look for opportunities to attack and finish points when your opponent is out of position.
- ✓ **Patience in defense**: Be patient and wait for the right moment to switch from defense to offense.

Fitness and stamina:
- ✓ **Stay fit**: Singles can be physically demanding, so maintain your fitness level to last through longer rallies.
- ✓ **Hydration**: Stay hydrated during matches to keep your focus and energy levels high.

Playing singles pickleball requires adaptability, quick decision-making, and physical stamina. Remember to cover the entire court effectively, maintain a balanced approach, and capitalize on opportunities to attack and defend. By mastering these basic strategies, you'll be on your way to becoming a formidable singles pickleball player. Enjoy the challenges and rewards that come with playing alone on the court!

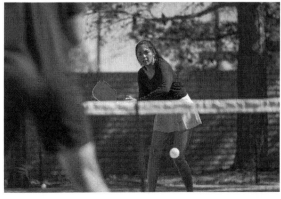

CHAPTER 7 DINKS, VOLLEYS AND LOBS

Welcome to **Chapter 7**. In this chapter, we explore the subtleties and skills required for dinking brilliance, mastering volley play, and executing effective lobs. Discover the art of the dink shot for control and placement, learn the techniques of net play mastery, and elevate your game with strategic lobbing techniques. Join us as we delve into Chapter 7 and unlock the secrets to these essential shots in pickleball.

7.1 DINKING BRILLIANCE: SUBTLE SHOTS FOR CONTROL AND PLACEMENT

Dinking is a highly strategic and nuanced aspect of pickleball that involves executing soft, controlled shots over the net from the Non-Volley Zone. This section delves into the technique, tactics, and key principles of dinking, helping you develop precise and strategic shots that can outmaneuver your opponents and dominate the game.

In pickleball, a **dink** refers to a soft and controlled shot where the ball is gently tapped over the net, aiming to keep it low and close to the net on the opponent's side. It involves delicately guiding the ball with finesse and touch, often executed with a short and compact swing. The purpose of a dink is to create precise placement, disrupt the opponent's positioning, and initiate strategic plays or set up opportunities for more aggressive shots.

Exploring the technique and tactics of dinking

Dinking requires a combination of touch, finesse, and precise placement. Here's a breakdown of the key elements:

- **Grip**: Hold the paddle with a relaxed grip, allowing for better touch and maneuverability.
- **Paddle angle**: Maintain a slightly upward angle on your paddle face to create a gentle trajectory and controlled contact with the ball.
- **Shot selection**: Observe your opponents' positioning and anticipate their reactions to choose the right shots, such as cross-court dinks or drop shots, to exploit weaknesses or create difficult angles.
- **Placement**: Aim for specific areas of the court, such as the sidelines, corners, or directly at your opponents' feet, to force them into defensive positions and limit their shot options.

Tips for executing precise and strategic dink shots

To enhance your dinking skills, consider the following tips:

- ✓ **Footwork**: Maintain a stable and balanced stance with your feet shoulder-width apart, enabling quick reactions and easy lateral movement along the Non-Volley Zone.

✓ **Soft touch**: Develop a delicate touch by using a combination of wrist and arm movement, focusing on finesse rather than power. Avoid excessive force that could result in hitting the ball too hard or long.

✓ **Timing**: Watch the ball closely and make contact at the optimal moment, just as it reaches the peak of its bounce. This allows you to control the speed, angle, and placement of your dinks.

✓ **Variation**: Incorporate different spin variations, such as topspin or backspin, to add deception and make it challenging for your opponents to anticipate the ball's trajectory.

Understanding the role of touch, angle, and placement in dinking exchanges

Dinking exchanges require a keen understanding of the role of touch, angle, and placement to gain an advantage over your opponents. Let's delve into the details:

Touch:
Developing a sensitive touch is essential in executing effective dink shots. It involves controlling the amount of force and spin applied to the ball to achieve the desired outcome. By practicing and fine-tuning your grip pressure and paddle angle, you can enhance your touch and manipulate the ball with precision.

Angle:
Utilizing angles effectively in dinking exchanges can create wider target areas and make it challenging for your opponents to anticipate and intercept your shots. Experiment with varying the angle of your dinks to exploit gaps in your opponents' positioning and create difficult shots for them to handle. Using acute angles can force your opponents to stretch and move out of position, opening up opportunities for follow-up shots or creating space for a winning shot.

Placement:
Strategic ball placement is crucial in dinking exchanges. Aim to keep the ball low and close to the net, forcing your opponents to hit up and limiting their ability to generate power. By placing the ball strategically, you can disrupt your opponents' rhythm, create opportunities to attack, and put them on the defensive. Target areas such as the sidelines, corners, or directly at your opponents' feet to exploit weaknesses and force difficult returns.

Incorporating touch, angle, and placement effectively in your dinking game can significantly impact the outcome of the rally. By mastering these aspects, you can control the pace, direction, and difficulty of your shots, keeping your opponents off balance and setting yourself up for success. Practice and refine your dinking skills to develop the finesse and precision required to execute accurate and strategic dinks consistently.

What are some **common mistakes beginners make** about the **dink** shot and what are some **tips to remedy** them?

Hitting the ball too hard: Beginners often make the mistake of hitting the dink shot too hard, resulting in the ball going out of bounds or providing an easy opportunity for the opponent to counterattack. **Remedy**: Focus on a soft touch and gentle swing, allowing the ball to drop close to the net and softly land in the opponent's Non-Volley Zone.

Lack of control: Beginners may struggle with controlling the direction and placement of their dink shots, leading to inconsistent and ineffective shots. **Remedy**: Practice controlling the angle and depth of your dink shots by adjusting your paddle face and using controlled wrist movement.

Poor footwork: Beginners sometimes neglect proper footwork when executing dink shots, resulting in off-balance and rushed shots. **Remedy**: Work on your footwork by maintaining a stable and balanced stance, stepping into the shot, and maintaining good court positioning.

Not utilizing spin: Beginners may overlook the importance of spin in dink shots, which can add variety and control to their shots. **Remedy**: Experiment with different spins, such as topspin or backspin, to influence the trajectory and bounce of the ball.

Inconsistent timing: Beginners often struggle with timing their dink shots, leading to mistimed swings and missed opportunities. Practice anticipating the ball's trajectory and adjust your timing accordingly, allowing the ball to drop to an optimal height before executing the shot.

Lack of patience: Beginners may rush their dink shots, trying to force the point or hit winners too quickly. Develop patience and focus on placement rather than power, aiming to keep the ball low over the net and making it difficult for the opponent to attack.

Failure to watch the ball: Beginners may lose sight of the ball during dink shots, resulting in mistimed shots and errors. **Remedy**: Keep your eye on the ball throughout the shot, focusing on its contact point with the paddle for better control and accuracy.

7.2 VOLLEY MASTERY: THE ART OF NET PLAY

In the game of pickleball, mastering the art of **volleying** at the net is crucial for maintaining control, dictating the pace of the game, and putting pressure on your opponents. This section will provide you with detailed instructions on techniques, positioning, timing, controlled touch, and strategic approaches to help you excel in volleying and dominate at the net.

In pickleball, a **volley** refers to hitting the ball in the air before it bounces on the court. It is a technique where the player strikes the ball while it is in flight, typically during close-range exchanges near the net. The volley requires quick reflexes, good hand-eye coordination, and precise control of the paddle.

The purpose of volleying is to maintain control and keep the ball in play during fast-paced rallies. By volleying, players can strategically place the ball and apply pressure on their opponents. It allows for quicker reactions and limits the time for opponents to respond, increasing the chances of winning the point.

Techniques for successful volleying at the net

First though, remember that in pickleball, the rule about volleying is known as the "two-bounce rule." According to this rule, there are specific restrictions on when players are allowed to volley the ball (hit it out of the air) without letting it bounce on the court.

The **two-bounce rule** states that both the serving team and the receiving team must let the ball bounce once on the court after the serve before they can start volleying. This means that the first shot, whether it's the return of serve or the serve itself, must be allowed to bounce before it can be volleyed.

After the initial bounce, players have the option to either volley the ball (hit it before it bounces) or let it bounce and play it as a groundstroke (hit it after it has bounced). From that point onward during the rally, players can choose to volley the ball or play it as a groundstroke as they see fit.

Mastering the art of volleying at the net is crucial for gaining an advantage in pickleball.

This section provides detailed instructions on the techniques that will help you execute successful volleys consistently and confidently.

Positioning:
✓ Stand near the net with your feet shoulder-width apart, maintaining a balanced and athletic stance.
✓ Position yourself slightly behind the kitchen line (Non-Volley Zone) to allow for quick reaction time and to cover a larger area.

Grip and racket preparation:
- ✓ Hold the racket (paddle) with a firm but relaxed grip, using a continental grip for versatility, control, and maneuverability.
- ✓ Position the paddle in front of your body, slightly above the wrist level, with the head facing slightly upwards to enable easy and quick paddle movement.

Footwork and movement:
- ✓ Stay on the balls of your feet to facilitate quick reactions and smooth movement.
- ✓ Utilize small shuffle steps or lateral movements to adjust your position as the ball approaches, ensuring you are always in an optimal position to make the volley.

Timing and contact point:
- ✓ Anticipate the incoming ball by closely observing your opponent's swing, body positioning, and the trajectory of the ball.
- ✓ Time your swing to make contact with the ball at the peak of its trajectory for better control and accuracy.

Controlled touch and placement:
- ✓ Use a compact swing and controlled touch to guide the ball over the net.
- ✓ Aim to keep the ball low and close to the net, making it challenging for opponents to counterattack and increasing the chances of a successful volley.

Importance of positioning, timing, and controlled touch in volley shots

Positioning, timing, and controlled touch play critical roles in executing effective volley shots. This section delves deeper into the significance of these factors and provides guidelines to help you maximize their impact on your game.

Positioning:
- ✓ Position yourself near the net, standing in an advantageous spot to intercept the ball and make effective volleys while staying clear of the kitchen area as per the rule.
- ✓ Continuously adjust your position in response to the angle and trajectory of the incoming shot, maximizing your chances of successfully executing volleys and maintaining control of the point.

A **reminder about volleying**: While positioning yourself near the net is advantageous, it's important to be mindful of the Non-Volley Zone, commonly known as the kitchen area. According to the rule, players are not allowed to volley the ball (hit it out of the air) while standing inside the kitchen. The kitchen is a 7-foot area on both sides of the net, and players must wait for the ball to bounce outside of the kitchen before they can enter and hit it in a volley.

By positioning yourself strategically near the net while also staying clear of the kitchen area, you can effectively control the game, respond to shots quickly, and set up opportunities to win points.

Timing:
✓ Anticipate the speed and direction of the ball to ensure proper timing for your volley.
✓ Be prepared to react quickly and adjust your positioning accordingly to meet the ball at the optimal moment.

Controlled touch:
✓ Focus on a soft and controlled touch when making contact with the ball.
✓ Use your wrist and forearm to absorb the ball's impact, maintaining a delicate touch for precise placement and controlled shots.

Strategies for attacking opponents' shots and maintaining control at the net

To dominate at the net, it is essential to develop effective strategies for attacking opponents' shots and maintaining control. This section provides valuable insights into these strategies, enabling you to seize opportunities and dictate the pace of the game.

Anticipation:
✓ Observe your opponents' positioning, shot patterns, and body language to anticipate their shots.
✓ Position yourself strategically to intercept and attack their shots effectively.

Angle and placement:
✓ Vary the angle and placement of your volleys to keep your opponents off-balance and guessing.
✓ Aim for areas of the court that force your opponents into difficult positions or create openings for winners.

Communication and collaboration (doubles play):
✓ Establish clear communication with your partner to coordinate shot selection and court positioning.
✓ Work together to cover the court efficiently, preventing gaps and maximizing control by anticipating each other's moves.

What are some **common mistakes beginners make** about the **volley** and what are some **tips to remedy** them?

Gripping the paddle too tightly: Beginners often grip the paddle too tightly during volleys, which can lead to a lack of control and finesse. **Remedy**: Relax your grip and hold the paddle with a firm but comfortable grip, allowing for better paddle maneuverability and touch.

Standing too far back: Beginners may position themselves too far back from the net during volleys, resulting in reaching or lunging for the ball and compromising balance and control. **Remedy**: Move closer to the net and maintain a balanced stance, allowing for easier and more controlled volley shots.

Incorrect paddle angle: Beginners sometimes hold the paddle at the wrong angle during volleys, leading to inconsistent shot direction and placement. **Remedy**: Keep the paddle face slightly open, allowing for a better angle to redirect the ball and control the shot trajectory.

Lack of anticipation: Beginners may react late to incoming volleys, leading to rushed shots and missed opportunities. **Remedy**: Work on anticipating the opponent's shot and be ready to react quickly, adjusting your position and preparing for the volley in advance.

Hitting the ball too hard: Beginners often make the mistake of trying to hit volleys with excessive power, resulting in the ball going out of bounds or into the net. **Remedy**: Focus on controlled and compact swings, focusing more on placement and accuracy rather than power.

Failure to move feet: Beginners may rely too much on arm movement during volleys and neglect footwork, limiting their ability to adjust to different ball positions. **Remedy**: Stay light on your feet and be ready to move quickly, using small steps to position yourself for optimal volleys.

Not keeping the ball low: Beginners may hit volleys with a high trajectory, giving opponents an opportunity to counterattack. **Remedy**: Aim to keep the ball low over the net, making it challenging for the opponent to make an effective return.

Lack of communication: Beginners playing doubles may struggle with communication during volleys, leading to confusion and missed shots. **Remedy**: Develop good communication with your partner, using clear signals or verbal cues to indicate who will take the volley and avoid collisions.

In pickleball, a **block** or **block volley** is a defensive shot that is performed near the net. It involves using a short and controlled motion to redirect the incoming ball back over the net without a full swing or follow-through.

The block is typically used in response to a hard-hit or fast-paced shot from the opponent, aiming to absorb the power of the ball and direct it back with accuracy and precision. The objective of the block is to return the ball over the net while keeping it low, making it challenging for the opponent to attack or counter the shot effectively. The block is executed with a firm yet relaxed grip on the paddle, allowing the player to quickly react and adapt to the speed and direction of the incoming shot. It requires good hand-eye coordination, timing, and anticipation of the opponent's shot.

The block is a valuable defensive technique in pickleball, enabling players to neutralize aggressive shots and maintain control of the rally.

By understanding and implementing these techniques, positioning, timing, controlled touch, and employing effective strategies, you will elevate your volleying.

7.3   LOBBING TECHNIQUES: ELEVATING YOUR SHOTS

The **lob** shot is a valuable technique in pickleball that can be a game-changer on the court. It involves hitting a high, arching shot that clears the opponents at the net and lands deep in the backcourt. In this section, we will explore the technique and strategy behind well-executed lobs, understand when and how to utilize them effectively, and provide tips for adjusting trajectory, power, and placement based on your opponents' positioning.

In pickleball, a **lob** refers to a high, arching shot that sends the ball deep into the opponent's court, aiming to go over their heads. The lob is executed by striking the ball with an upward trajectory, imparting significant height and minimal forward power.

The lob serves as a defensive or strategic shot, often used to counter aggressive opponents who are positioned close to the net. By hitting a well-placed lob, players can force their opponents to retreat towards the baseline, buying themselves time to reposition and regain control of the point.

Exploring the technique and strategy behind well-executed lobs

The lob shot is a powerful tool in your arsenal that allows you to regain control, change the pace of the game, and disrupt your opponents' rhythm. In this section, we will delve into the technique and strategy behind the lob shot, enabling you to incorporate it into your game effectively.

Grip and racket (paddle) preparation:
✓ Use a semi-western or eastern backhand grip for better control and range of motion.
✓ Position the paddle head slightly open, allowing for an upward swing path to generate height and distance on the lob.

Footwork and positioning:
✓ Position yourself further back from the net to create the necessary angle and height for the lob.
✓ Utilize small shuffle steps or a crossover step to adjust your positioning and set up the ideal launching point for the lob.

Swing mechanics:
✓ Initiate your swing with a smooth and controlled motion, gradually accelerating the paddle.
✓ Focus on making contact with the ball slightly below its center, using a brushing motion to generate backspin and height.

Trajectory and placement:
✓ Aim for a high, arching trajectory that clears the opponents at the net and lands deep in the backcourt.
✓ Target areas of the court that force your opponents into a defensive position or create difficult angles for them to attack.

Understanding when and how to utilize lobs effectively

The lob shot can be a game-changer when used strategically. Knowing when and how to incorporate lobs into your gameplay is essential for gaining an advantage on the court. In this section, we will explore the situations where the lob shot can be most effective and provide guidance on its effective utilization.

Opponent positioning:
✓ Use the lob when your opponents are positioned close to the net or are expecting a low, hard shot.
✓ The lob disrupts their rhythm, forces them to retreat, and creates opportunities for you to regain control of the point.

Defensive situations:
✓ Employ the lob shot when you are out of position or facing an aggressive shot from your opponents.
✓ The lob buys you time to recover, reset the point, and regain control of the game.

Court awareness:
✓ Assess the court dimensions, wind conditions, and your opponents' strengths and weaknesses before attempting a lob.

By considering these factors, you can determine the most effective placement and trajectory for your lob shot.

Tips for adjusting trajectory, power, and placement based on opponents' positioning

Adapting your lob shot to your opponents' positioning is crucial for maximizing its effectiveness. In this section, we will provide tips for adjusting the **trajectory**, **power**, and **placement** of your lob shot based on your opponents' positioning on the court.

Trajectory:
✓ Consider the height and angle of your lob shot to exploit your opponents' positioning.
✓ A higher trajectory allows you to clear opponents at the net and land the ball deep in the backcourt, making it more challenging for them to retrieve.

Power:
✓ Adjust the power of your lob shot to disrupt your opponents' rhythm and control the pace of the game.
✓ Vary the power of your lobs based on your opponents' proximity to the net and their ability to retrieve high shots effectively.

Placement:
✓ Aim for strategic placement of your lobs to create difficulties for your opponents.
✓ Target areas such as the corners, sidelines, or gaps in their court coverage to force them into uncomfortable positions and limit their shot options.

By skillfully adjusting the trajectory, power and placement of your lob shots, you can keep your opponents on their toes, exploit their weaknesses, and gain an advantage on the court.

CHAPTER 8   OVERHEADS AND TRANSITION PLAY

Welcome to **Chapter 8** of our pickleball guide, where we delve into the exciting world of overhead shots and transition play. In this chapter, we will explore the art of overhead dominance, focusing on the powerful and strategically placed smash shots that can elevate your game to new heights. We will also delve into the tactics and techniques of transition area play, mastering the art of resets and positioning. Get ready to take your pickleball skills to the next level as we uncover the secrets of overheads and transition play, providing you with the knowledge and tools to become a formidable force on the court.

8.1   OVERHEAD DOMINANCE: SMASHING SHOTS FOR POWER AND PLACEMENT

In the context of pickleball, the **smash** and the **overhead shot** are often used interchangeably. Both terms refer to a powerful shot executed with an overhead motion, where the player strikes the ball forcefully downward. The smash/overhead shot is typically employed when the ball is high, allowing the player to generate maximum power and drive the ball aggressively towards the opponent's side of the court. It is a dynamic offensive shot that aims to create a difficult return for the opponent and gain a tactical advantage in the rally.

The overhead shot is often used to hit the ball downwards with speed and intensity, aiming to place it in an advantageous position on the opponent's side of the court. This shot requires good timing, footwork, and technique to ensure a successful execution.

Mastering the overhead shot can significantly enhance a player's offensive capabilities and provide opportunities to dominate rallies and dictate the pace of the game.

Mastering the technique and mechanics of overhead shots

Mastering the overhead shot is crucial for adding power and precision to your game. In this section, we will explore the key techniques and mechanics to help you achieve mastery in your overhead shots.

Positioning and preparation:
✓ Position yourself under the ball with your feet shoulder-width apart and your non-dominant foot slightly forward.
✓ Hold the paddle with a continental grip for optimal control and power.

Timing and contact point:
✓ Anticipate the ball's trajectory by watching your opponent's shot and adjust your positioning accordingly.
✓ Time your swing to make contact with the ball at the highest point of its arc.

Generating power and accuracy:
- ✓ Engage your legs, core, and upper body to generate power in your overhead shots.
- ✓ Rotate your hips and shoulders while maintaining a stable base to transfer energy into the shot.
- ✓ Follow through with your swing, extending your arm and wrist for accuracy and control.

Generating power and accuracy in overhead smashes

Overhead smashes are explosive shots that can catch your opponents off guard. In this section, we will delve into the techniques that will help you generate maximum power and accuracy in your overhead smashes.

Body mechanics and weight transfer:
- ✓ Bend your knees and load your legs to generate power.
- ✓ Transfer your weight from your back foot to your front foot as you swing to maximize power.
- ✓ Snap your wrist at the point of contact to add extra speed and spin to the ball.

Timing and ball contact:
- ✓ Watch the ball closely and time your swing to make contact at the highest point.
- ✓ Extend your arm fully to reach the ball and make a clean contact with the center of the paddle.

Strategies for placing overhead shots effectively in different game situations

Placing your overhead shots effectively can give you a significant advantage on the court. In this section, we will explore various strategies that will help you place your overhead shots precisely and strategically in different game situations.

Court awareness and shot selection:
- ✓ Assess the court and your opponents' positioning to identify open areas.
- ✓ Choose your target based on your opponents' weaknesses or areas where they are less likely to reach the ball.

Targeting weaknesses:
- ✓ Aim your overhead shots towards your opponents' weaker side or areas where they struggle to defend effectively.
- ✓ Exploit their vulnerabilities by placing the ball out of their reach or creating difficult angles.

Varying shot selection:

✓ Mix up your overhead shots by using different variations, such as flat smashes, angled smashes, and drop smashes.

✓ Adjust the trajectory, power, and placement of your shots based on the specific game situation and your opponents' positions.

Top tips:

What are some **common mistakes beginners make** about **overhead shots** and what are some **tips to remedy** them?

Poor timing: Beginners often struggle with timing their overhead shots, resulting in mistimed swings and missed opportunities. Remedy: Practice tracking the ball's trajectory and anticipate its descent to time your swing correctly.

Incorrect grip: Using the wrong grip on overhead shots can lead to inconsistent and less powerful shots. **Remedy**: Ensure you have a proper continental grip, where your hand is positioned in a way that allows for optimal control and power during overhead shots.

Insufficient leg drive: Beginners may neglect to utilize their legs effectively when executing overhead shots, leading to weaker shots and reduced power. **Remedy**: Focus on initiating the shot with a strong leg drive, pushing off the ground to generate upward momentum and power in your swing.

Lack of shoulder rotation: Beginners often overlook the importance of shoulder rotation in overhead shots, resulting in limited power and accuracy. **Remedy**: Practice rotating your shoulders as you swing, using your upper body to generate power and direct the shot effectively.

Overcomplicating the shot: Some beginners may overthink the overhead shot, causing hesitation and inconsistency. **Remedy**: Simplify the shot by focusing on a smooth and fluid swing motion, keeping your eye on the ball, and trusting your instincts.

Failure to track the ball: Beginners may struggle with tracking the ball during overhead shots, which can lead to mistimed swings and missed opportunities. **Remedy**: Practice following the ball's flight path from the opponent's shot to ensure better timing and accuracy in your overhead shots.

Lack of practice: Overhead shots require practice to develop consistency and confidence. **Remedy**: Dedicate time to practicing overhead drills, focusing on technique, footwork, and timing, to improve your overhead shot proficiency.

8.2   TRANSITION AREA TACTICS: MASTERING RESETS AND POSITIONING

In pickleball, the transition area plays a vital role in regaining control and setting up advantageous positions on the court. In this section, we will delve into the techniques and strategies that will help you master resets and positioning in the transition area.

Understanding the importance of the transition area in pickleball

The **transition area**, often referred to as the "no man's land," is the region between the Non-Volley Zone and the baseline. Understanding the significance of this area is key to taking advantage of opportunities during transition play. Let's explore the techniques and tactics that will elevate your game in the transition area.

Anticipation and readiness:
✓ Stay alert and anticipate the ball's trajectory as it approaches the transition area.
✓ Position yourself optimally to be ready for quick reactions and decisive shots.
✓ Focus on reading your opponents' body language and racket (paddle) positioning to anticipate their shots.

Court awareness:
✓ Develop a keen sense of court awareness by constantly scanning the court, assessing your opponents' positions, and identifying open spaces.
✓ Understand the geometry of the court and identify high-percentage target areas where you can place your shots effectively.

Techniques for resetting the ball and regaining control during transition play

Resetting in pickleball refers to the act of returning the ball to a neutral position during transition play. It involves executing shots such as soft shots, lobs, or high percentage shots, with the intention of regaining control and disrupting your opponents' momentum. The purpose of resetting is to create an opportunity to regain a favorable position on the court. Resetting shots are characterized by controlled touch, strategic placement, and thoughtful decision-making. By neutralizing the point and potentially shifting the momentum in your favor, resetting allows you to set up the next shot or exploit your opponents' vulnerabilities.

In this section, we will delve into the techniques and strategies that will enhance your ability to execute effective resets and maximize your performance during transition play.

Soft shots and dinks:
✓ Utilize soft shots, such as dinks and drop shots, to reset the ball and bring it back to a neutral position.
✓ Focus on controlled touch and placement rather than power to keep your opponents off balance.
✓ Aim for the corners of the court to make it difficult for your opponents to reach the ball.

Lobs:
✓ Employ lobs as a reset option when your opponents are too close to the net or crowding the transition area.

✓ Aim for deep and high lobs to buy time and create space for yourself or your partner to recover.
✓ Vary the trajectory and placement of your lobs to keep your opponents guessing and make it challenging for them to execute strong returns.

High percentage shots:
✓ Opt for high percentage shots, such as cross-court drives or deep groundstrokes, to reset the ball with consistency and minimize unforced errors.
✓ Focus on hitting with good depth and control, targeting areas of the court where your opponents are less likely to attack.
✓ Keep the ball away from the middle of the court, as it allows your opponents to easily transition from defense to offense.

Positioning strategies to optimize court coverage and capitalize on opportunities in the transition area

Positioning in the transition area is a crucial aspect of pickleball that can greatly impact your ability to capitalize on opportunities and maintain control of the game. In this section, we will explore effective positioning strategies that will help you optimize your court coverage and make the most of transition play.

Splitting the court:
One key positioning strategy is to split the court, which involves placing yourself and your partner in a way that covers different areas of the court. By splitting the court, you create a larger defensive and offensive coverage area, making it more challenging for your opponents to find open spaces to exploit. This positioning also allows for effective communication and coordination with your partner.

Anticipation and reaction:
Anticipate your opponents' shots by reading their body language, racket (paddle) positioning, and court positioning. React quickly to their shots by moving efficiently and smoothly to the appropriate position on the court. Anticipating and reacting effectively will help you cover more ground and be prepared for incoming shots, enabling you to maintain control during the transition.

Maintaining depth and angle:
Position yourself in a way that maintains proper depth and angle on the court. Stay close to the kitchen line to defend against short shots and be ready to move forward for volleys. At the same time, maintain a position that allows you to cover the deeper areas of the court and handle deep shots effectively. Adjust your positioning based on the speed and trajectory of the incoming shot to optimize your court coverage.

Communication and teamwork:
Effective communication and coordination with your partner are essential in transition play. Constantly communicate with your partner about your

positioning, shots, and any potential opportunities or threats on the court. Work together to ensure seamless transitions between defensive and offensive positions, allowing you to maintain control and take advantage of openings in your opponents' defense.

Controlled placement: When transitioning from defense to offense, focus on placing your shots strategically. Look for open areas on the court, target weak spots in your opponents' positioning, and aim for shots that are difficult to retrieve. By placing your shots with control and precision, you can maintain an offensive advantage and put pressure on your opponents.

Exploiting opportunities: Be alert to opportunities that arise during transition play. Capitalize on weak shots from your opponents by attacking aggressively and taking control of the rally. Look for openings in your opponents' court coverage or moments of hesitation and take advantage of them with well-placed shots. Stay proactive and ready to seize opportunities to maintain momentum in the game.

By implementing these positioning strategies and techniques, you can optimize your court coverage, capitalize on opportunities in the transition area, and maintain control of the game. Practice these strategies in your pickleball matches to become a formidable force during transition play and elevate your overall performance on the court.

CHAPTER 9   BACKHAND EXCELLENCE

Welcome to **Chapter 9** of our book, where we dive into the realm of backhand excellence in pickleball. In this chapter, we will focus on enhancing your skills and strategies to improve your weak side, the backhand. Whether you're new to the game or an experienced player looking to refine your technique, we have you covered. We will explore various aspects of the backhand shot, including breakthrough strategies to overcome common challenges, mastering the two-handed backhand for added power and stability, and unleashing the elegance and finesse of the one-handed backhand. Get ready to elevate your game and unlock the full potential of your backhand as we delve into the techniques, tactics, and secrets of backhand excellence in pickleball.

9.1   BACKHAND BREAKTHROUGH: STRATEGIES TO IMPROVE YOUR WEAK SIDE

The **backhand** is a crucial shot in pickleball, utilizing the non-dominant side of your body to strike the ball. Unlike the forehand, where the dominant hand leads the way, the backhand relies on your non-dominant hand for execution. It plays a vital role in reaching balls on the opposite side of your body and maintaining control and versatility on the court.

The backhand refers to a shot executed with the non-dominant hand on the side of the body opposite to the hand holding the paddle. It is a stroke where the player strikes the ball using the backside or the top side of the paddle, depending on the technique employed. The backhand requires proper footwork, timing, and hand-eye coordination to generate power, control, and spin while maintaining balance and stability on the court. Mastering the backhand allows players to effectively return shots hit to their weak side, execute precise shots, and be well-rounded and versatile on the pickleball court.

The term **weak side** refers to the non-dominant side of a player, which in the context of pickleball, is the side opposite to their dominant hand. Strengthening your weak side, particularly your backhand, is vital for achieving a balanced skillset and creating a well-rounded game. By dedicating time and effort to improve your backhand stroke, you will gain a competitive edge and enhance your ability to handle various shot scenarios effectively.

Techniques for developing a strong backhand stroke

Look at the following techniques for developing a strong backhand stroke:

Grip and hand placement:
✓ Establish a proper grip on the paddle, such as the continental grip, which offers stability and control for backhand shots.
✓ Position your non-dominant hand comfortably on the paddle, ready to provide support and stability.

Body positioning:
- ✓ Adopt an **athletic stance** with a slight bend in your knees, ensuring a solid base for generating power and maintaining balance.
- ✓ Position yourself with your shoulders parallel to the net, allowing for an optimal swing.

Swing mechanics:
- ✓ Focus on a compact and controlled swing for better accuracy and consistency.
- ✓ Initiate the swing by rotating your hips and shoulders, transferring your weight from the back foot to the front foot.
- ✓ Keep the swing path straight and on the same plane, maintaining a relaxed grip and fluid motion.

Follow-through:
- ✓ Complete your backhand stroke with a full and extended follow-through.
- ✓ Let your paddle finish high, pointing towards your target, to ensure accuracy and power in your shots.

Drills and exercises to enhance backhand control and power

Here are some drills and exercises to enhance backhand control and power:

- ✓ **Shadow swings**: Stand in front of a mirror or imagine an opponent, and practice your backhand stroke. Pay attention to maintaining proper technique, body positioning, and a smooth follow-through.
- ✓ **Wall hits**: Stand a few feet away from a wall and hit the ball against it using your backhand. This drill helps improve control as you observe the ball's trajectory and adjust your stroke accordingly.
- ✓ **Live ball drills**: Engage in drills with a partner or practice in game-like scenarios to simulate real-match situations. Work on hitting consistent backhand shots, responding to different ball placements, and adjusting your footwork and positioning.

Strategies for incorporating the backhand into your game plan

Here are some strategies for incorporating the backhand into your game plan:

- ✓ **Identifying opportunities**: Recognize situations where using the backhand can give you an advantage, such as reaching wide shots, countering opponents' cross-court shots, or returning shots with topspin or slice.
- ✓ **Court coverage**: Develop court awareness and positioning to ensure you are well-prepared for backhand shots. Anticipate and move efficiently to cover the backhand side of the court, allowing you to handle incoming shots with confidence.
- ✓ **Shot selection**: Practice different types of backhand shots, including drives, volleys, drops, and lobs. Learn to assess the situation and choose the appropriate shot based on factors like the ball's height, speed, and your position on the court.

✓ **Targeted practice**: Dedicate specific practice sessions to focus on your backhand stroke. Work on improving consistency, accuracy, and power by targeting specific areas of the court and varying the pace and placement of your shots.

Top tips:

What are some **common mistakes beginners make** about the **backhand** and what are some **tips to remedy** them?

Gripping the paddle too tightly: Beginners often grip the paddle too tightly during backhand shots, which can restrict their wrist movement and accuracy. **Remedy**: Ensure a relaxed grip, allowing for more fluid wrist action and better control over the shot.

Using excessive force: Beginners may try to generate power on their backhand by using excessive force, resulting in inconsistent shots and loss of control. **Remedy**: Instead, focus on using proper technique and timing to generate power, emphasizing a smooth and controlled swing.

Poor body positioning: Lack of proper body positioning can lead to ineffective backhands. Beginners may find themselves off-balance or too far from the ball, making it challenging to execute a strong backhand. **Remedy**: Work on maintaining a balanced and athletic stance, positioning yourself well to anticipate and reach the ball comfortably.

Inadequate preparation: Beginners often fail to prepare early for backhand shots, leading to rushed and uncontrolled swings. **Remedy**: Ensure proper footwork, getting in position early, and using a compact backswing to prepare for the shot.

Neglecting follow-through: Some beginners may neglect the follow-through on their backhand, resulting in inconsistent shots and reduced power. **Remedy**: Practice a complete follow-through, extending the paddle towards the target after making contact with the ball, to improve consistency and generate more power.

Lack of practice: Backhand shots require dedicated practice to develop consistency and confidence. **Remedy**: Regularly practice backhand drills, focusing on technique, footwork, and timing, to improve your backhand skills over time.

9.2   MASTERING THE TWO-HANDED BACKHAND

The **two-handed backhand** is a fundamental stroke in pickleball that involves using both hands on the grip to strike the ball on your non-dominant side. It offers several advantages, including enhanced stability, control, and power, making it a valuable shot in your repertoire. In this section, we will delve into the fundamentals of the two-handed backhand grip and technique, explore its advantages and disadvantages, and provide tips for refining your two-handed backhand to increase consistency.

Understanding the fundamentals of the two-handed backhand grip and technique

✓ **Grip**: Hold the paddle with a continental grip, placing your dominant hand on the bottom of the handle and your non-dominant hand above it, creating an overlapping grip. This grip allows for better stability and control during the stroke.

✓ **Stance and body positioning**: Stand with your feet shoulder-width apart, knees slightly bent, and body positioned sideways with your non-dominant side facing the net. This stance helps optimize your balance and allows for efficient weight transfer during the stroke.

✓ **Backswing**: Rotate your shoulders and torso sideways, turning your non-dominant side towards the net. Keep your arms extended and maintain a relaxed grip on the paddle. The backswing prepares your body for generating power and sets the foundation for a smooth swing.

✓ **Swing path and contact point**: Swing forward smoothly, aiming to make contact with the ball in front of your body, slightly ahead of your front foot. Maintain focus on the ball throughout the swing to ensure clean and solid contact.

✓ **Follow-through**: After making contact with the ball, extend your arms fully and follow through towards your target. This complete follow-through helps generate power and control, directing the ball with precision.

Advantages and disadvantages of the two-handed backhand

Let's look at the advantages and disadvantages of the two-handed backhand.

Advantages of the two-handed backhand:

• **Enhanced stability**: The use of both hands on the grip provides increased stability and control, allowing for better shot placement and accuracy.
• **Increased power:** The additional support from the non-dominant hand helps generate more power in the shot, allowing for stronger and more aggressive strokes.
• **Versatility**: The two-handed grip allows for easier manipulation of the paddle face, providing versatility in generating different types of spin (topspin, slice, and flat shots) and adapting to various playing conditions.

Disadvantages of the two-handed backhand:

• **Limited reach**: The two-handed backhand may limit your reach compared to a one-handed backhand, making it more challenging to stretch and reach balls outside your hitting zone. It is important to adjust your positioning and footwork accordingly.
• **Reduced flexibility**: Using both hands on the grip can restrict the flexibility and range of motion in your wrist, potentially limiting your ability to generate certain types of shots or make quick adjustments.

Tips for refining the two-handed backhand and increasing consistency

Practice drills:
Incorporate specific **drills** targeting your two-handed backhand, such as cross-court and down-the-line shots, or repetitive stroke development against a wall. These drills help improve your muscle memory and reinforce proper technique.

Muscle memory:
Develop **muscle memory** by practicing your two-handed backhand regularly. Muscle memory refers to the ability of your muscles to remember and repeat specific movements without conscious thought. Focus on repetition and quality practice to ingrain the proper mechanics.

Footwork and positioning:
Work on your footwork to ensure proper positioning and body alignment when executing the two-handed backhand. Good footwork helps generate power and maintain balance. Practice moving into the optimal position for each shot, adjusting your stance based on the ball's trajectory and your desired shot selection.

Video analysis:
Record and analyze your two-handed backhand technique to identify areas for improvement. Seek feedback from a coach or experienced player to refine your stroke. Compare your technique to professional players to understand the key elements of an effective two-handed backhand.

Adaptability:
Adapt your two-handed backhand technique based on court position, ball trajectory, and opponent's shot. Develop the ability to adjust and respond to various playing conditions. Practice hitting different types of shots, such as **defensive slices**, **offensive topspins**, and **neutral flat shots**, to expand your shot repertoire and adapt to different game situations.

By following these detailed instructions and dedicating focused practice to your two-handed backhand, you can develop a strong and reliable stroke. Regular repetition, analysis, and adjustment will contribute to improving your two-handed backhand and increasing your consistency on the pickleball court.

9.3   UNLEASHING THE ONE-HANDED BACKHAND

The **one-handed backhand** is a versatile and elegant stroke in pickleball that involves using a single hand on the grip to strike the ball on your non-dominant side. While the two-handed backhand is commonly used, the one-handed backhand offers its own advantages, including increased reach, versatility, and potential for greater power. In this section, we will explore the mechanics of the one-handed backhand stroke, provide instructions for developing proper footwork and body positioning, and offer strategies for generating power and precision with the one-handed backhand.

Exploring the mechanics of the one-handed backhand stroke

Grip and hand position:
Adopt a continental grip or an eastern grip to provide better control and maneuverability for the one-handed backhand. Place your non-dominant hand below the grip to stabilize the paddle.

Swing path and racket (paddle) preparation:
Initiate the swing with a semi-circular motion, bringing the racket (paddle) back early and keeping it high to create a longer swing path. Maintain a relaxed grip and a slightly open stance.

Upper body rotation and follow-through:
Engage your core and rotate your upper body to generate power and transfer energy into the shot. Ensure a full follow-through, extending your arm and racket (paddle) towards the target.

Developing proper footwork and body positioning for the one-handed backhand

Stance and balance:
Begin with a shoulder-width stance and maintain a balanced position throughout the stroke. Bend your knees slightly to maintain stability and generate power.

Footwork and preparation:
Anticipate the incoming shot and move into the ideal position early. Use a split-step to stay light on your feet and be ready to adjust and react to the ball's trajectory.

Body alignment and weight transfer:
Position your body perpendicular to the net, with your non-dominant shoulder facing the target. Transfer your weight forward into the shot by pushing off your back foot.

Strategies for generating power and precision with the one-handed backhand

Timing and contact point:
Time your swing so that you make contact with the ball in front of your body, slightly off-center towards the non-dominant side. Aim to hit the ball at the optimal height to maximize power and control.

Body rotation and hip rotation:
Rotate your hips and shoulders towards the net as you swing, generating rotational power and adding pace to your shot. This rotation also helps in maintaining control and accuracy.

Control and touch:
Practice developing control and touch with your one-handed backhand by incorporating drop shots, lobs, and angled shots into your training. Focus on the finesse and accuracy of your strokes to vary the pace and placement of your shots.

By understanding the mechanics, developing proper footwork and body positioning, and implementing effective strategies, you can unleash the full potential of your one-handed backhand.

Dedicate focused practice to these instructions, and with time and repetition, you will refine your technique, increase your power and precision, and confidently execute the one-handed backhand on the pickleball court.

CHAPTER 10   DETECTING OUT BALLS

Detecting **out balls** is crucial in pickleball as it ensures fair play and maintains the integrity of the game. Importantly, look at where the ball lands! Making accurate calls on whether a ball is in or out impacts the flow of the game, determines the outcome of points, and can greatly influence the strategies employed by players. By having the ability to detect out balls, players can maintain a level playing field, promote sportsmanship, and prevent disputes on the court. It is an essential skill that allows for fair and competitive gameplay.

The determination of whether a ball is out relies on accurate observation, analysis of its flight trajectory, and assessment of the bounce patterns. Making the correct call on out balls is essential for maintaining fairness and ensuring that the game is played within the established rules and boundaries.

10.1   ANALYZING BALL FLIGHT: UNDERSTANDING TRAJECTORY AND SPIN

Being able to accurately analyze the flight of the ball is a crucial skill that can greatly impact your performance and decision-making on the court. By understanding the concepts of **trajectory** and **spin**, you can gain valuable insights into how the ball moves through the air and how it will behave upon contact with the court. This knowledge allows you to anticipate the ball's path, make better shot selections, and improve your overall gameplay.

Understanding trajectory – predicting the path

Understanding the **trajectory** of the ball is essential in pickleball as it allows you to anticipate where the ball will land on the court. By analyzing the flight path of the ball, you can position yourself more effectively, giving you a competitive advantage in gameplay.

To effectively analyze ball flight in pickleball, it's important to understand the different types of trajectory and how to adjust your gameplay accordingly. Here are some key points to consider:

High trajectory:
This refers to shots that are hit with a higher arc, causing the ball to travel higher over the net. High trajectory shots are often used to clear opponents and create depth in the court. To handle high trajectory shots, position yourself closer to the baseline, maintain a balanced stance, and be prepared to move quickly to track the ball.

Flat trajectory:
A flat trajectory means the ball is hit with minimal arc, resulting in a faster and more direct shot. Flat shots are commonly used for quick and aggressive plays, such as drives and smashes. To handle flat shots, react quickly, maintain a low and balanced stance, and use your reflexes to return the ball with precision.

Low trajectory:
Low trajectory shots are hit with a lower arc, close to the net. These shots are typically used for dinks and drop shots, aiming to keep the ball low and close to the net, making it difficult for opponents to return. When facing low trajectory shots, be ready to bend your knees, stay close to the net, and use soft hands to control the ball and execute a well-placed return.

Arched trajectory:
An arched trajectory involves hitting the ball with a high, looping arc. This type of shot is often used for lobs, where the aim is to send the ball high over the opponent and land it deep in their court. When facing arched trajectory shots, track the ball carefully, adjust your positioning towards the baseline, and be prepared to move swiftly to track and return the ball.

Deep shots:
Deep shots refer to shots that are hit towards the back of the court, close to the baseline. These shots aim to push opponents deeper into their court and create opportunities for offensive plays. When facing deep shots, position yourself towards the baseline, move quickly to track the ball, and execute a well-placed return to regain control of the point.

Short shots:
Short shots are hit close to the net, aiming to catch opponents off guard and force them to move forward quickly. These shots require precise control and delicate touch. When facing short shots, be prepared to move close to the net, maintain a low and balanced stance, and use soft hands to guide the ball over the net and land it in a challenging position for your opponent.

Angle of descent:
The angle at which the ball descends after crossing the net is an important aspect to consider when analyzing ball flight. Shots with a steeper angle of descent tend to drop faster, making them more challenging to return. To handle shots with a steep angle of descent, adjust your positioning and footwork accordingly, anticipate the ball's trajectory, and be ready to move quickly to reach and return the shot.

Understanding spin - deciphering the effects

When detecting out balls, understanding the spin can provide valuable clues to determine whether a shot is in or out. Here's how observing the spin can help in detecting out balls:

Rotation:
The rotation of the ball in the air can affect its trajectory. For example, a shot with topspin tends to have a more pronounced downward trajectory, making it more likely to stay in bounds. Conversely, a shot with backspin may have a higher bounce and a shorter distance, potentially resulting in an out ball.

Bounce:
Different spin effects can influence the ball's bounce after it hits the ground. Backspin can cause the ball to bounce lower and potentially go out, while topspin can generate a higher bounce that keeps the ball in play. By observing the bounce, you can gauge whether the ball has stayed within the court boundaries.

Flight path:
The spin applied to the ball can alter its flight path. Sidespin, for instance, can make the ball curve or veer off its expected trajectory. By carefully tracking the ball's flight, you can detect any deviation from a straight line, indicating a possible out ball.

Speed:
The spin on the ball can affect its speed. Shots with topspin may have a faster pace, while shots with backspin can slow down. If a shot appears unusually fast or slow compared to what you expected, it may be an indicator of an out ball.

Contact point:
Observing the point of contact between the ball and the paddle can provide insights into the intended spin. Players typically make adjustments in their paddle angle and contact point to generate specific spin effects. By noticing where the player strikes the ball, you can infer the type of spin and evaluate whether it might result in an out ball.

By paying attention to these spin-related factors - rotation, bounce, flight path, speed, and contact point - you can better assess whether a shot is in or out. Remember to rely on your observations and understanding of spin to make more accurate out calls during pickleball matches.

10.2   OBSERVING BALL BOUNCE PATTERNS: IDENTIFYING IN OR OUT

Reading the bounce

Here are some tips:

- ✓ Pay close attention to the height and speed of the ball as it bounces on the court. A higher and faster bounce typically indicates that the ball has landed inside the court boundaries, while a lower and slower bounce may suggest that the ball has landed out.
- ✓ Observe the angle at which the ball bounces off the surface. If the ball bounces at a sharp angle or deviates significantly from the expected path, it could be an indication that the ball has landed out.
- ✓ Look for irregular or unpredictable bounces that deviate from the normal trajectory. A ball that bounces erratically or unpredictably may have hit the net or an obstacle, resulting in it being out of bounds.
- ✓ Take note of any excessive spin or sideways movement that affects the bounce. Spin can influence the direction and trajectory of the ball, causing it to veer off its intended path. If the ball exhibits excessive spin that takes it outside the court boundaries, it should be considered out.

✓ Assess the consistency of the bounce across different areas of the court. If you notice that the ball consistently bounces differently in certain areas of the court, it could indicate that those areas have uneven or irregular playing surfaces, affecting the accuracy of the ball's landing.

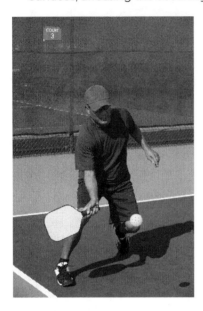 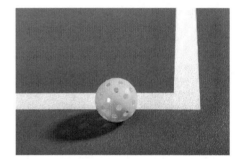

Analyzing the patterns

Here are some tips:

✓ Identify common bounce patterns that indicate whether the ball is likely to be in or out. For example, if you consistently observe that balls hit with a specific type of shot tend to bounce a certain way when they are out of bounds, you can use that pattern to help you make accurate calls.
✓ Observe how the ball reacts to different shots and strokes played by both you and your opponent. By paying attention to how the ball behaves after specific shots, you can gain valuable insights into whether the ball has landed in or out of the court.
✓ Look for trends or tendencies in the bounce patterns that can help you make accurate calls. For instance, if you notice that balls hit with a powerful topspin tend to stay within the court boundaries, while balls hit with a slice tend to bounce out, you can use this knowledge to judge the ball's location more effectively.
✓ Take into account the height, speed, and angle of the shot that precedes the bounce. The characteristics of the shot can influence the bounce of the ball. By considering the shot's trajectory and power, you can make better judgments about whether the ball has landed in or out.
✓ Pay attention to the positioning and movement of your opponent to gauge their judgment on the ball's location. If your opponent reacts as if the ball is out of bounds, it can provide additional evidence to support your decision.

✓ Practice and familiarize yourself with different bounce patterns through regular gameplay and observation. The more experience you gain in observing and interpreting bounce patterns, the more confident and accurate you will become in detecting whether a ball is in or out of bounds.

10.3   MAKING ACCURATE CALLS: IMPROVING YOUR JUDGMENT

Making accurate calls requires focus, observation, and practice. By following these instructions, you can enhance your judgment and contribute to a fair and enjoyable pickleball experience for all players.

Focus on the ball:
✓ Maintain a clear and unobstructed line of sight to the ball at all times. Keep your eyes on the ball from the moment it leaves your opponent's paddle until it lands.
✓ Position yourself in a way that allows you to see the ball's trajectory and landing spot as accurately as possible. Adjust your stance and positioning on the court accordingly.
✓ Avoid distractions and stay mentally focused on the ball. Minimize external factors that can interfere with your judgment, such as crowd noise or movements.
✓ Train your eyes to track the ball's movement effectively. Practice following the ball's path during drills and gameplay to improve your visual tracking skills.

Use the right perspectives:
✓ Utilize your best vantage points to judge the ball's location accurately. Find positions on the court that provide you with the clearest view of the ball's landing area.
✓ Move quickly and efficiently to get into the optimal position to make the call. Anticipate where the ball is heading and position yourself accordingly to get a better perspective.
✓ When in doubt, use different angles and perspectives to confirm your judgment. If you are unsure about the ball's location, try to move to a different position on the court to get a different view.

Trust your instincts:
✓ Develop a sense of timing and intuition to anticipate the ball's landing. Pay attention to the speed, trajectory, and spin of the shot to make an informed judgment.
✓ Trust your initial instinct when making a call. Your initial reaction is often based on your subconscious assessment of the ball's location.
✓ Refrain from making assumptions or biased judgments based on personal interests or favoritism. Strive to be impartial and make decisions solely based on your observation and assessment of the ball's landing.

Communicate effectively:
- ✓ Use clear and concise language when making a call. Announce your decision confidently and audibly, ensuring that your opponent and any onlookers can hear your call.
- ✓ Be respectful and open to discussions or challenges from your opponent. Engage in a respectful dialogue to resolve any disagreements or uncertainties regarding the call.
- ✓ Seek the assistance of a third party if necessary. If you and your opponent are unable to reach a consensus on a call, consult a referee or another neutral party to make a final ruling.

Continuously improve:
- ✓ Learn from your experiences and seek feedback from fellow players or coaches. Reflect on your judgment calls and analyze any areas for improvement.
- ✓ Practice making accurate calls during training sessions and friendly matches. Simulate game situations and actively assess the ball's location to enhance your judgment skills.
- ✓ Stay updated with the rules and regulations of pickleball to ensure that your judgment aligns with the official guidelines. Regularly review the rules and seek clarification if needed.

CHAPTER 11   FITNESS AND INJURY PREVENTION

In **Chapter 11**, we delve into the important aspects of fitness and injury prevention in the context of pickleball. As an active and dynamic sport, pickleball requires players to be physically prepared and resilient to avoid injuries and enhance their performance on the court. In this chapter, we will explore the essential elements of warm-up routines that help prepare your body for peak performance, ensuring that you are ready to give your best during gameplay. Additionally, we will discuss valuable tips and strategies for injury prevention and conditioning, enabling you to stay in the game and enjoy pickleball with confidence and longevity. Let's embark on a journey of fitness and injury prevention, enhancing our well-being and taking our pickleball skills to new heights.

11.1   WARM-UP ESSENTIALS: PREPARING FOR YOUR PEAK PERFORMANCE

Warm-ups are essential pre-exercise routines designed to prepare the body for physical activity. They typically consist of a series of dynamic movements and exercises that gradually increase the heart rate, warm up the muscles, and improve flexibility and range of motion.

Importance of warm-up exercises and stretches in preventing injuries

Warm-ups serve several important purposes. Firstly, they help to increase blood flow to the muscles, which improves oxygen and nutrient delivery, enhancing muscle performance. Secondly, warm-ups increase body temperature, making the muscles more pliable and less prone to injury. Additionally, warm-ups activate the nervous system, improving coordination, reaction time, and overall motor skills. By engaging in a proper warm-up routine, players can optimize their physical readiness, reduce the risk of injury, and perform at their best during pickleball matches.

In addition to the physical benefits, warm-ups also have a psychological aspect that should not be overlooked. They help players mentally prepare for the upcoming activity, allowing them to shift their focus and concentrate on the game ahead. Warm-ups provide an opportunity to mentally rehearse movements, strategies, and game plans, fostering a sense of readiness and confidence. They can also serve as a transition from the distractions of daily life to the present moment, creating a focused and present mindset.

In the context of pickleball, **stretches** refer to specific exercises or movements that aim to elongate and loosen the muscles and tendons in the body. These stretching exercises are performed before and after playing pickleball to improve flexibility, increase range of motion, and prevent muscle tightness and injury. Stretching can target various muscle groups involved in pickleball, such as the shoulders, arms, legs, and core. It helps to prepare the body for physical activity by gradually increasing blood flow, warming up the muscles, and improving their elasticity. Stretching in pickleball is an essential component of a well-rounded warm-up routine and can contribute to better performance, enhanced agility, and reduced risk of strains or sprains.

By incorporating warm-up essentials into their routine, players can optimize their performance, reduce the risk of injuries, and approach each game with a prepared body and a focused mind. It is a crucial step in ensuring peak performance and enjoying the game to its fullest.

Tips for warm-up exercises and stretches

Dynamic movements:
Dynamic movements are active and rhythmic exercises that involve the major muscle groups and help increase blood circulation, warm up the body, and prepare the muscles and joints for physical activity. Examples include:

✓ **Arm circles**: Stand with your feet shoulder-width apart and extend your arms to the sides. Make circular motions with your arms, gradually increasing the size of the circles.
✓ **Leg swings**: Stand next to a wall or support and swing one leg forward and backward in a controlled manner, keeping the rest of your body stable.
✓ **Torso twists**: Stand with your feet shoulder-width apart and rotate your upper body from side to side, allowing your arms to swing naturally with the movement.
✓ **Hip rotations**: Stand with your feet hip-width apart and rotate your hips in a circular motion, as if you're hula hooping.

Cardiovascular exercises:
Cardiovascular exercises are activities that elevate the heart rate, increase blood circulation, and warm up the entire body. They are important to improve cardiovascular fitness, enhance endurance, and prepare the body for physical exertion. Examples of cardiovascular exercises for warm-up include:

✓ **Jogging in place**: Lift your knees and pump your arms as you jog on the spot.
✓ **Jumping jacks**: Stand with your feet together and your arms by your sides. Jump and simultaneously spread your legs out to the sides while raising your arms above your head.
✓ **Jump rope**: Use a skipping rope and jump over it while maintaining a steady rhythm.

Dynamic stretches:
Dynamic stretches are active stretching exercises that involve moving parts of your body through a full range of motion. These stretches are performed in a controlled and deliberate manner, mimicking the movements used in pickleball. Dynamic stretches help warm up the muscles, increase their flexibility, and prepare the body for the dynamic movements required during the game. They are different from static stretches as they involve continuous movement instead of holding a stretch for an extended period. Examples of dynamic stretches for warm-up include:

- ✓ **Walking lunges**: Take a step forward with your right foot and lower your body into a lunge position, ensuring your right knee is directly above your ankle. Push off with your right foot and bring your left foot forward, repeating the motion as you walk.
- ✓ **High knee marches**: Stand tall and march in place while lifting your knees as high as possible, trying to bring them up to hip level. Maintain a good posture and engage your core muscles throughout the movement.
- ✓ **Arm swings**: Extend your arms straight out to the sides and swing them forward and backward in a controlled motion. Gradually increase the range of motion as you warm up.

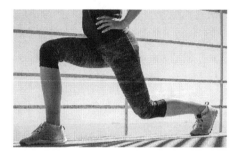

Specific muscle activation:
Specific muscle activation exercises target the muscles used in pickleball and help activate them before the game. These exercises engage the major muscle groups, improve joint mobility, and enhance readiness for action. Examples of specific muscle activation exercises include:

- ✓ **Squats**: Stand with your feet shoulder-width apart and lower your body by bending your knees and pushing your hips back, as if you're sitting in a chair. Keep your chest up and your weight on your heels. Push through your heels to return to the starting position. Squats engage the leg muscles, including the quadriceps, hamstrings, and glutes.
- ✓ **Plank**: Start in a push-up position with your forearms resting on the ground and your body in a straight line. Engage your core muscles and hold this position for a set amount of time. Planks activate the core muscles, including the abdominals, obliques, and lower back, which are crucial for stability and balance during pickleball.

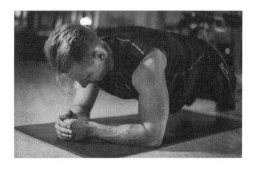

✓ **Shoulder rotations**: Stand tall with your arms relaxed at your sides. Lift your arms to the sides and rotate them forward in small circles. Gradually increase the size of the circles. Shoulder rotations activate the shoulder muscles, including the deltoids and rotator cuff muscles, which are involved in various pickleball shots.

The importance of gradual progression:
Gradually progress through your warm-up routine, starting with lighter intensity exercises and gradually increasing the intensity as your body warms up. This allows your muscles, joints, and cardiovascular system to adjust to the increasing demands. By paying attention to your body's response, you can adjust the warm-up duration and intensity based on your individual needs, minimizing the risk of injury and preparing optimally for the game.

Customizing warm-up routines to meet your specific needs

Customizing warm-up routines to meet your specific needs means tailoring your pre-game warm-up to address your individual requirements, areas of tightness, muscle imbalances, and previous injuries. By doing so, you can ensure that your body is properly prepared for the game of pickleball.

This customization involves assessing your body, focusing on specific stretches that target your areas of concern, addressing any muscle imbalances, modifying dynamic movements to suit your limitations, and incorporating personalized exercises or drills that benefit your game.

By customizing your warm-up routine, you can optimize your performance, reduce the risk of injuries, and enhance your overall experience on the pickleball court. It is recommended to seek guidance from a fitness professional or coach to help identify specific areas of focus and tailor exercises to your needs.

When it comes to warming up before a game of pickleball, it's important to tailor your routine to meet your specific needs. Everyone's body is unique, and different individuals may have varying areas of tightness, muscle imbalances, or previous injuries. By customizing your warm-up routine, you can address these specific needs and ensure that your body is properly prepared for the game. Here are some tips for customizing your warm-up routine:

Assess your body:
Before starting your warm-up, take a moment to assess your body and identify any areas that feel tight or require attention. Pay attention to any previous injuries or areas of chronic discomfort. This assessment will help you determine which areas need extra focus during your warm-up.

Focus on specific stretches:
Incorporate stretches that target the areas of your body that require attention. For example, if you have tight hamstrings, include hamstring stretches in your routine. If you have shoulder issues, add specific shoulder stretches to improve mobility and flexibility in that area.

Address muscle imbalances:
If you have identified muscle imbalances, such as one side of your body being stronger or more flexible than the other, include exercises that help correct these imbalances. This may involve additional stretching or strengthening exercises for specific muscle groups.

Modify dynamic movements:
Adjust the intensity and range of motion of your dynamic movements to suit your needs. If you have any joint limitations or mobility issues, modify the movements to ensure they are safe and effective for your body. For example, if you have knee issues, perform smaller, controlled movements during lunges or squats.

Incorporate personalized exercises:
Consider incorporating personalized exercises or drills that directly benefit your pickleball game. This may include footwork drills, agility exercises, or specific shot practice. By focusing on these aspects, you can enhance your game-specific skills and improve your overall performance.

Remember, the goal of customizing your warm-up routine is to address your unique needs and ensure that your body is properly prepared for the demands of pickleball. Pay attention to any discomfort or limitations and adjust your routine accordingly.

It's important to consult with a fitness professional or a coach if you need guidance on identifying specific areas of focus or modifying exercises. By customizing your warm-up routine, you can optimize your performance, reduce the risk of injuries, and enjoy a more enjoyable and successful game of pickleball.

11.2   STAYING IN THE GAME: INJURY PREVENTION AND CONDITIONING TIPS

In this section, we will explore valuable strategies and tips for **injury prevention** and **conditioning** in pickleball. Injury prevention is crucial to ensure a safe and enjoyable playing experience, while conditioning plays a vital role in enhancing performance and maintaining optimal physical fitness. By implementing effective injury prevention techniques and incorporating conditioning strategies into your training routine, you can minimize the risk of injuries, improve your overall fitness, and elevate your game on the pickleball court. Let's delve into these essential aspects of staying in the game: injury prevention and conditioning tips.

Injury prevention strategies

Injury prevention in pickleball refers to the strategies and practices implemented to minimize the risk of injuries during gameplay. It involves taking proactive measures to protect your body and maintain physical well-being. By following proper techniques, adopting safety precautions, and addressing common injury-prone areas, you can reduce the likelihood of sustaining injuries and enjoy a safer and more enjoyable pickleball experience.

Warm-up and cool-down:
Begin each session with a thorough **warm-up** routine, as discussed in the previous section, to prepare your muscles, joints, and cardiovascular system for the demands of the game. Similarly, incorporate a **cool-down** phase at the end of play to gradually reduce intensity and promote recovery.

Proper technique:
Focus on using correct form and technique in your shots and movements. This includes using the appropriate body mechanics, maintaining good posture, and executing shots with proper alignment. Seek guidance from experienced players or coaches to ensure you are using proper technique and minimizing the risk of injury.

Protective gear:
Consider using protective gear, such as knee pads, elbow braces, or wrist supports, to provide additional support and stability to vulnerable areas of your body. Wearing supportive footwear with adequate cushioning and ankle support is also important.

Listen to your body:
Pay attention to any pain, discomfort, or signs of overexertion during play. It is crucial to listen to your body and take breaks when needed. Ignoring warning signs can lead to more serious injuries.

Conditioning tips for peak performance

Conditioning in pickleball refers to the physical preparation and training necessary to enhance overall fitness, strength, endurance, and agility. By focusing on specific conditioning exercises and incorporating them into your training routine, you can improve your performance, reduce the risk of injuries, and maintain a high level of play.

Strength training:
Include exercises that target the major muscle groups involved in pickleball, such as the legs, core, and upper body. This can include exercises like squats, lunges, planks, push-ups, and rows. Strengthening these areas helps improve stability, power, and control during gameplay.

Endurance training:
Enhance your cardiovascular fitness through activities like running, cycling, or swimming. Building endurance allows you to sustain a high level of performance throughout a game or match without fatigue.

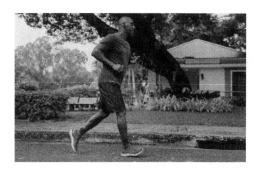

Agility and quickness drills:
Incorporate drills that focus on improving your footwork, reaction time, and change of direction. This can involve ladder drills, cone drills, or shuttle runs. Agility training enhances your ability to move swiftly and efficiently on the court.

Flexibility and mobility exercises:
Dedicate time to stretching and mobility exercises to improve joint range of motion and reduce the risk of muscle imbalances. Incorporate dynamic stretches, as discussed earlier, to promote flexibility and prepare the body for dynamic movements during play.

Rest and recovery:
Adequate rest and recovery are essential components of conditioning. Allow your body sufficient time to recover between training sessions and matches to prevent overuse injuries and optimize performance.

Nutrition and hydration:
Maintain a balanced and nutritious diet to support your overall health and performance. Adequate hydration is also crucial for optimal physical functioning and injury prevention. Stay hydrated by drinking water before, during, and after play.

Cross-training:
Engage in cross-training activities that complement your pickleball training. This can include activities like yoga, Pilates, or strength training exercises that target different muscle groups and enhance overall fitness.

Recovery strategies:
Incorporate effective recovery strategies into your routine, such as foam rolling, stretching, and massage therapy. These techniques help reduce muscle soreness, improve flexibility, and promote faster recovery between training sessions.

Gradual progression:
Gradually progress your training intensity, duration, and difficulty level to avoid overloading your body and risking injuries. Allow ample time for adaptation and avoid sudden increases in training volume or intensity.

Monitoring and assessment:
Regularly monitor your progress and assess your performance to identify areas for improvement. This can involve keeping a training log, tracking your stats, or seeking feedback from coaches or training partners.

Consultation with professionals:
If you have specific concerns, pre-existing injuries, or unique training goals, it is advisable to consult with healthcare professionals, sports trainers, or qualified coaches. They can provide personalized guidance, injury management strategies, and training recommendations based on your individual needs.

Top tips:

In pickleball, a **hydration break** refers to a designated pause in the game to allow players to hydrate and rehydrate themselves. These breaks are important to prevent dehydration and maintain optimal performance on the court.

In social or casual games, hydration breaks can be taken as needed or whenever players feel the need to hydrate. There are no strict rules or regulations regarding the timing and duration of these breaks. Players can take a break during changeovers or at any suitable moment during the game.

In tournaments, the use of hydration breaks may vary depending on the tournament rules and conditions. Some tournaments may schedule specific time intervals for hydration breaks, typically after a certain number of games or at set intervals during longer matches. The duration of the breaks is usually limited to a few minutes to ensure the smooth flow of the tournament.

Hydration breaks are particularly crucial in hot and humid conditions to prevent heat-related illnesses and maintain player safety. It is essential for players to stay properly hydrated throughout the game to maintain their performance, endurance, and overall well-being.

It is recommended that players bring their own water bottles or hydration packs to the court and take advantage of the hydration breaks to replenish fluids and electrolytes.

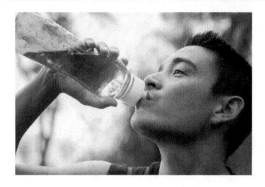

By following these injury prevention and conditioning tips, you can optimize your physical readiness, reduce the risk of injuries, and improve your overall performance in pickleball. Remember that every individual is unique, and it's essential to listen to your body, adapt your training to your specific needs, and seek professional guidance when necessary. Prioritizing injury prevention and conditioning will contribute to your long-term health, enjoyment, and success in the game of pickleball.

CHAPTER 12 EMBRACING FAIR PLAY AND ENJOYING THE GAME

In the world of pickleball, the values of good sportsmanship and fair play are integral to fostering a positive and enjoyable playing environment. This chapter delves into the importance of these principles and explores how they shape the essence of the game.

12.1 PLAYING WITH RESPECT: EMBRACING GOOD SPORTSMANSHIP AND FAIR PLAY

By embracing **good sportsmanship**, players cultivate a culture of respect, camaraderie, and inclusivity on and off the court. Upholding **fair play** ensures that the game is conducted with integrity, fairness, and equal opportunities for all. What do these concepts look like on the pickleball court? Let's dive into the sub-sections that highlight the significance of good sportsmanship and fair play in the world of pickleball.

Embracing good sportsmanship

In the game of pickleball, **good sportsmanship** is a vital aspect that goes beyond the physical skills and strategies. It encompasses a set of values and behaviors that create a positive and supportive environment for all players involved. Good sportsmanship is about more than just winning or losing; it's about playing with integrity, respect, and fairness towards both your opponents and teammates.

In casual games, demonstrating good sportsmanship means approaching each match with a positive attitude. It involves showing kindness and encouragement to fellow players, regardless of their skill level. Whether you win or lose, it's important to maintain a gracious and humble demeanor, acknowledging the efforts and achievements of others. Good sportsmanship in casual games also means exhibiting good manners on and off the court, such as saying "good game," shaking hands, and expressing appreciation for your opponents' efforts.

In more formal settings, such as tournaments or competitive leagues, good sportsmanship involves adhering to the rules and regulations set forth by the governing bodies. It means respecting the decisions of officials and accepting them without argument. It also means exhibiting a high level of sportsmanlike conduct throughout the entire event, both in victory and defeat. This includes acknowledging your opponents' skill, celebrating their successes, and showing empathy and support when they encounter challenges.

Upholding fair play

Fair play is a fundamental principle in pickleball that ensures equal opportunities, integrity, and a level playing field for all participants. Upholding fair play means adhering to the established rules and regulations, playing honestly, and demonstrating a sense of fairness in every aspect of the game.

In casual games, upholding fair play means making accurate line calls and respecting the boundaries of the court. It means acknowledging your mistakes and correcting any unintentional rule violations. Treating your opponents with respect and considering their perspectives is also an essential part of fair play. It's important to recognize that everyone is there to enjoy the game and have a fair chance to succeed.

In more formal competitions, upholding fair play extends beyond rule adherence. It encompasses ethical behavior, respect for officials, and graciousness towards opponents. It means accepting both victories and defeats with dignity and displaying sportsmanlike conduct throughout the entire competition. Fair play involves recognizing the importance of honest competition and valuing the integrity of the game over personal gains.

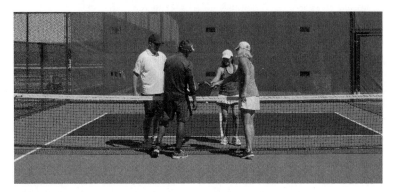

12.2   PICKLEBALL ETIQUETTE

Etiquette is a set of unwritten rules that govern social behavior, ensuring respect, consideration, and fairness among individuals. In the context of pickleball, etiquette plays a crucial role in maintaining a positive and enjoyable atmosphere on the court. It emphasizes the importance of good sportsmanship, communication, and respect for opponents, partners, and fellow players. By practicing pickleball etiquette, players create an environment where everyone can fully engage in the game, fostering a sense of camaraderie and fair play. Etiquette not only enhances the overall experience of playing pickleball but also contributes to the growth and reputation of the sport as a whole.

Pre-match:

✓ Warmly greet other players: Introduce yourself and ask your opponents if they have any questions or concerns.
✓ Ask for permission before joining a game: Wait until the point is over to ask permission to join and wait until the next game starts if necessary.
✓ Arrive on time: Show up at least 10 minutes early to warm up and stretch.

During the match:

✓ Avoid making excessive noise: Keep your voice level low, avoid yelling or cursing, and be mindful of your body movements.
✓ Communicate with your partner: Use hand gestures or verbal cues to coordinate plays with your partner and avoid collisions.
✓ Respect the court boundaries: Step away from the net when your opponents are hitting the ball, and don't go over the line when serving or returning the serve.
✓ Do not touch the net: Avoid making contact with the net or grabbing it during gameplay.
✓ Allow the ball to bounce: Let the ball bounce once on your side of the court before hitting it back over the net.

End of the match:

✓ Shake hands with your opponents: Thank your opponents for playing and congratulate them on their game.
✓ Help clean up the court: Collect any stray balls, water bottles, or other debris, and dispose of them properly.
✓ Show respect for your fellow players: Don't argue about points or calls and avoid confrontational behavior.
✓ Congratulate the winning team: Acknowledge your opponents' skill and congratulate them on their victory.
✓ Avoid gloating if you win: Be gracious in victory and avoid rubbing your opponents' loss in their faces!

Other tips:

✓ Avoid using foul language: Curse words or derogatory terms can offend other players and detract from the game.
✓ Bring your own equipment: Don't borrow a paddle or other equipment without asking first, and make sure your paddle meets pickleball standards.
✓ Wait for a clear court before entering: Avoid walking onto the court during play and wait until the ball is dead to enter or exit.
✓ Stay hydrated: Bring a water bottle or sports drink to stay hydrated, especially in hot or humid weather.
✓ Be mindful of other players' health and safety: If a player falls or appears injured, pause the game to check on them and help if needed.
✓ Follow court-specific rules: Observe signs or markings on the court, and respect any special rules or guidelines set by the facility or organization.

CHAPTER 13   TAKING YOUR SKILLS TO THE NEXT LEVEL

In **Chapter 13**, we focus on providing valuable insights and tips to help both beginning players and more experienced players elevate their game. For beginners transitioning to an intermediate level, we offer essential advice on how to improve and progress in their skills. For more experienced players looking to reach new heights, we delve into mastering advanced techniques to enhance their performance. Additionally, we explore strategic gameplay strategies to develop tactical awareness on the court. Lastly, we emphasize the importance of mental toughness and provide guidance on building a winning mindset, fostering confidence, and resilience. This chapter aims to empower players at all levels to continue their journey of improvement and take their pickleball skills to new levels of proficiency.

13.1   TRANSITIONING FROM BEGINNER TO INTERMEDIATE: ESSENTIAL TIPS FOR IMPROVEMENT

As a beginner player transitioning to the intermediate level, there are several essential tips that can help you improve your skills and elevate your game.

- ✓ Firstly, focus on developing a strong foundation of fundamental techniques such as proper grip, footwork, and paddle control. Work on refining your strokes, including the serve, forehand, backhand, and dinks. Practice consistency and accuracy in your shots, gradually increasing the power and speed as you gain more confidence.
- ✓ Another important aspect of transitioning to the intermediate level is expanding your knowledge of the game. Study the rules, strategies, and scoring system in detail to understand the nuances of pickleball.
- ✓ Take the time to analyze your gameplay and identify areas that need improvement. Work on your court awareness, anticipation, and positioning to enhance your overall game sense.
- ✓ Additionally, seek opportunities to play with and learn from more experienced players. Participate in clinics, workshops, or join local pickleball groups to engage with a diverse range of players. Playing against stronger opponents challenges you and pushes you to elevate your skills.

Remember to maintain a positive mindset and embrace the learning process. Improvement takes time and effort, so be patient with yourself and celebrate small victories along the way. Consistent practice, dedication, and a growth mindset will help you make a successful transition from beginner to intermediate level.

13.2   MASTERING ADVANCED TECHNIQUES: TAKING YOUR GAME TO NEW HEIGHTS

For more experienced players looking to take their game to new heights, mastering advanced techniques is crucial.

- ✓ Focus on honing your skills in areas such as power shots, spin variations, and advanced footwork.
- ✓ Develop a more versatile and aggressive style of play to keep your opponents off balance.
- ✓ Work on adding more spin to your shots, such as topspin, backspin, and sidespin, to add variety and control to your game.
- ✓ Experiment with different grips and paddle angles to achieve the desired spin effects.
- ✓ Additionally, practice advanced shots like the lob, drop shot, and overhead smash to expand your shot repertoire.
- ✓ Advanced footwork is another key aspect of elevating your game. Improve your agility, speed, and lateral movement to cover more ground on the court. Focus on efficient weight transfer, quick direction changes, and explosive movements to reach difficult shots and maintain optimal court positioning.

To take your game to the next level, analyze and strategize your gameplay. Develop a deeper understanding of shot selection, court coverage, and opponent analysis.

Adapt your tactics based on the strengths and weaknesses of your opponents and be prepared to adjust your game plan during matches.

Lastly, continue to challenge yourself by participating in competitive events and tournaments. Test your skills against high-level players and learn from the experience. Embrace the opportunity to compete and grow as a player.

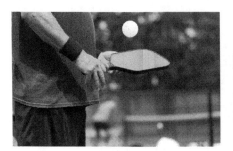
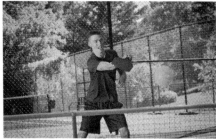

13.3 ELEVATING STRATEGIC GAMEPLAY: TACTICAL APPROACHES FOR SUCCESS

Strategic gameplay is a vital component of pickleball at any level. To elevate your game strategically, focus on understanding the dynamics of the game and implementing effective tactics. Analyze the strengths and weaknesses of your opponents and develop a game plan accordingly.

One key tactic is to vary your **shot selection** and placement. Mix up your shots with a combination of dinks, drives, lobs, and drop shots to keep your opponents guessing and off balance. Aim for the open areas of the court and exploit your opponents' vulnerabilities.

Court positioning is another crucial aspect of strategic gameplay. Learn to anticipate your opponent's shots and position yourself optimally to cover the court effectively.

Maintain proper spacing with your partner during doubles play and communicate effectively to ensure seamless coordination.
Developing a strong defense is equally important. Master the art of blocking shots and returning difficult balls. Focus on positioning yourself well to retrieve shots effectively and maintain a solid defensive posture.

Lastly, adaptability is a key attribute in strategic gameplay. Be prepared to adjust your tactics and game plan based on the flow of the match. Stay mentally engaged, analyze your opponent's patterns, and make necessary adjustments to gain the upper hand.

By elevating your strategic gameplay, you can gain a competitive edge and increase your chances of success on the pickleball court.

13.4 DEVELOPING MENTAL TOUGHNESS: BUILDING CONFIDENCE AND RESILIENCE

Developing mental toughness is crucial for taking your pickleball skills to the next level. Building confidence and resilience can help you stay focused, overcome challenges, and perform at your best, especially in competitive situations.

One important aspect of mental toughness is maintaining a **positive mindset**. Cultivate self-belief and confidence in your abilities. Visualize success and affirm your skills and strengths. Develop strategies to manage negative thoughts and emotions, such as self-doubt or frustration, and maintain a calm and composed demeanor on the court.

Resilience is another key component of mental toughness. Learn to bounce back from setbacks or mistakes and maintain a resilient attitude. Use failures or losses as opportunities for learning and growth, rather than dwelling on them negatively.

Develop coping mechanisms and techniques, such as deep breathing, visualization, or positive self-talk, to regain focus and composure during challenging moments.

Effective goal setting is also essential for mental toughness. Set specific, achievable goals that align with your skill level and desired outcomes. Break down your larger goals into smaller, manageable steps and track your progress along the way. Celebrate milestones and accomplishments to boost your confidence and motivation.

Building mental toughness also involves developing effective routines and rituals. Create pre-game rituals that help you enter a focused and positive state of mind. This may include visualization exercises, warm-up routines, or specific breathing techniques. Establish a routine for handling pressure situations, such as taking a moment to regroup and refocus before important points or matches.

Maintaining a strong support system is crucial for mental toughness. Surround yourself with positive and supportive individuals who believe in your abilities and provide encouragement. Seek guidance from coaches, mentors, or sports psychologists who can offer strategies to enhance your mental resilience.

Lastly, cultivate a growth mindset that embraces challenges and values the learning process. Embrace setbacks as opportunities for improvement and see them as valuable experiences that contribute to your growth as a player. Approach each practice and match with a mindset of continuous improvement, focusing on learning and developing new skills.

By developing mental toughness, you can enhance your performance, handle pressure situations effectively, and elevate your overall gameplay. Building confidence, resilience, and a positive mindset will not only impact your performance on the pickleball court but also in other areas of your life.

FINAL THOUGHTS: REFLECTING ON YOUR PICKLEBALL JOURNEY

As you reach the final pages of this book, it's time to reflect on your pickleball journey and celebrate the progress you've made. Whether you're a beginner just starting out or a seasoned player looking to take your skills to new heights, you have embarked on an exciting and fulfilling adventure in the world of pickleball.

Throughout this book, we have explored the fundamentals, strategies, and techniques that will help you become a more confident and skilled player. From mastering the basic shots to understanding game tactics, from developing mental toughness to improving physical conditioning, you have gained valuable insights and tools to enhance your game.

But beyond the technical aspects, pickleball is about so much more. It's about the joy of stepping onto the court, the camaraderie with fellow players, and the sense of accomplishment with each improvement. It's about the laughter, the challenges, and the unforgettable moments shared with friends old and new.

As you continue your pickleball journey, remember to embrace the spirit of the game. Approach each practice session, each match, and each tournament with a positive mindset and a love for the sport. Cherish the friendships you've made along the way and the memories created on the court. Stay open to learning and growing, as there is always more to discover in this dynamic and evolving sport.

Whether you play for recreation, competition, or both, pickleball has the power to bring people together, foster personal growth, and create lifelong connections. As you continue to hone your skills, never lose sight of the joy and passion that drew you to the game in the first place.

So, as you close this book, take a moment to reflect on how far you've come and the exciting possibilities that lie ahead. Remember that your pickleball journey is unique and personal, and it will continue to unfold in its own remarkable way.

Thank you for joining us on this pickleball adventure. We hope that this book has inspired and empowered you to excel in the game you love. Now, go out there, enjoy every moment on the court, and continue to write your own incredible pickleball story.

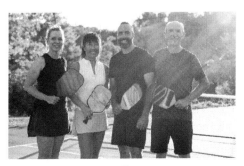

APPENDIX – QUICK REFERENCE GUIDE
SCORING AND RULES SUMMARY

THE BASIC RULES
#1 The pickleball game, and each point, begins with a serve
#2 In pickleball, we have an underhand serve, or a drop serve, and that serve must go cross court
#3 After the serve, each point continues until there is a fault
#4 You can hit groundstrokes in the kitchen, but you can't volley while in the kitchen
#5 The ball must bounce on both sides before either team can volley
#6 Only the serving team can score points

The server must call loudly before each serve. Before each serve, the server must call the serve so that other players on the pickleball court hear and know the score. The server should call the score loudly prior to hitting the pickleball on serve.

In **singles pickleball**, the score is made up of **two numbers** (for example, **0-0**). The first number represents the server's score (**0**). The second number represents the receiver's score (**0**). There isn't a third number because, in singles pickleball, each side has only one rather than two serves. For example, if the score in singles pickleball is **8-6**, this means that the server has **8 points**, and the receiver has **6 points**.

In **doubles pickleball**, the score is made up of **three numbers** (for example, **0-0-2**). The first number represents the serving team's score (**0**). The second number represents the receiving team's score (**0**). The third number represents the server number, either **#1** or **#2**. For example, if the score in doubles pickleball is **8-6-2**, this means that the serving team has **8 points**, the receiving team has **6 points**, and the serving team is on **player #2**.

Basic line call rules – "in" or "out"?

Shots on the lines of the pickleball court are "**in**", with one exception – the Non-Volley Zone line on the serve is "**out**".

The basic pickleball **line call rules** are:

- The pickleball must land in the correct service court on the serve. All of the lines of the correct service court, except for the Non-Volley Zone line (kitchen line) are "**in**". So, if the service pickleball lands on the sideline, centerline or baseline, the serve is "**in**". If the pickleball serve lands in the Non-Volley Zone, on the Non-Volley Zone line, or completely outside of the lines of the service court, then the serve is "**out**".

- On any shot, other than the serve, the pickleball in "**in**" if it lands anywhere on the pickleball court. This includes all of the lines of the pickleball court. So, if the pickleball lands on the sideline, centerline, baseline, or the Non-Volley Zone line on any shot, other than the serve, then the pickleball is "**in**." If the pickleball lands completely outside of the lines on the pickleball court, then the pickleball is "**out**."
- If the pickleball is "**in**", the rally continues on. If the pickleball is "**out**", then the player (singles) or team (doubles) that hit the pickleball out of bounds would have committed a fault and loses the rally.

"**Out**" calls are made by the pickleball players on the side of the pickleball court where the pickleball bounces.

If the pickleball hits you (other than below your wrist, such as your finger), then you lose the rally.

THE MUST KNOW SINGLES PICKLEBALL SCORING RULES
#1 The first serve for each side begins on the right-hand/even side
#2 If the server wins the point, the server will switch sides of the court
#3 If the receiver wins the rally, neither player switches sides of the court and there will be a side out
#4 The server keeps the serve until the server loses the rally
#5 If the server loses the rally, then the serve goes to the receiver

THE MUST KNOW DOUBLES PICKLEBALL SCORING RULES
#1 The first serve for each side begins on the right-hand/even side
#2 If the serving team wins the point, the server will switch sides and serve from the other side of the court
#3 If the receiving team wins the rally, then the serve goes to the second server on the serving team
#4 The server keeps the serve until the server loses the rally
#5 If the serving team loses the rally, then the serve goes to the second server or the receiving team (if applicable)

Note: In doubles pickleball, the server switches sides with their partner after each point. This means that the server will alternate serving from the right and left sides of the court. For example, if the first server starts serving from the right side of the court and wins the point, they will then switch sides with their partner and serve from the left side of the court for the next point. If they win that point as well, they will switch back to the right side of the court to serve again. This pattern continues until the serving team loses a rally, at which point the serve goes to the second server on the serving team or to the first server on the receiving team, if applicable.

It's important to note that players do not switch sides with their partner when they are receiving. The receiving team stays on their respective sides of the court until they win a rally and gain the serve.

PICKLEBALL RATINGS AND RANKINGS

USAPA ratings summary

1.0–2.0	A player who is just starting to play pickleball and has no other sports background.
2.5	A player who has limited experience and can sustain a short rally.
3.0	A player who understands fundamentals and court positioning.
3.5	A player who can understand the difference between a hard game and a soft game. They move quickly to the Non-Volley Zone. They understand when stacking may be effective.
4.0	A player who is able to identify and attack their opponents' weaknesses. They are aware of their partners' position on the court and are able to move as a team.
4.5	A player who understands strategy and has good footwork. They are able to communicate and move well with their partner.
5.0	A player who has mastered pickleball strategies. They have efficient footwork and can easily adjust their game to their opponents' strengths and weaknesses. They rarely make unforced errors.
5.5+	A player who has mastered pickleball. They are a top-caliber player.

USAPA Player Skill Ratings

self-rating score	self-rating guideline
1.0-2.0	This player is just starting to play pickleball and has no other sports background. Minimal understanding of rules of the game.

self-rating score	self-rating guideline
2.5	• This player has minimal experience. • Can sustain a short rally with players of equal ability. • Basic ability to keep score.

self-rating score	self-rating guideline
3.0	**FOREHAND:** Ability to hit a medium-paced shot. Lacks directional intent and consistency. **BACKHAND:** Avoids using backhand. Lacks directional intent and consistency. **SERVE/RETURN:** Able to hit a medium paced shot. Lacks depth, direction, and consistency. **DINK:** Not able to consistently sustain a dink rally. Not yet developed the ability to control this shot. **3RD SHOT:** Generally hits a medium paced shot with little direction. **VOLLEY:** Able to hit a medium paced shot. Lacks direction/inconsistent. **STRATEGY:** Understands fundamentals. Is learning proper court positioning. Knows the fundamental rules and can keep score and is now playing tournaments.

self-rating score	self-rating guideline
3.5	**FOREHAND**: Improved stroke development with moderate level of shot control. **BACKHAND**: Learning stroke form and starting to develop consistency but will avoid if possible. **SERVE/RETURN**: Consistently gets serve/return in play with limited ability to control depth. **DINK**: Increased consistency, with limited ability to control height/depth. Sustains medium length rallies. Starting to understand variations of pace. **3RD SHOT**: Developing the drop shot in a way to get to the net. **VOLLEY**: Is able to volley medium paced shots thereby developing control. **STRATEGY**: Moves quickly towards the Non-Volley Zone (NVZ) when opportunity is there. Acknowledges difference between hard game and soft game and is starting to vary own game during recreation and tournament play. Can sustain short rallies. Is learning proper court positioning. Basic knowledge of stacking and understands situations where it can be effective.

self-rating score	self-rating guideline
4.0	**FOREHAND**: Consistently hits with depth and control. Is still perfecting shot selection and timing. **BACKHAND**: Has improved stroke mechanics and has moderate success at hitting a backhand consistently. **SERVE/RETURN**: Places a high majority of serves/returns with varying depth and speed. **DINK**: Increased consistency with moderate ability to control height/depth. May end dink rally too soon due to lack of patience. Is beginning to understand difference between attackable balls and those that are not. **3RD SHOT**: Selectively mixing up soft shots with power shots to create an advantage with inconsistent results. **VOLLEY**: Able to volley a variety of shots at different speeds. Is developing consistency and control. Starting to understand the block/re-set volley. **STRATEGY**: Aware of partner's position on the court and is able to move as a team. Demonstrates ability to change direction in an offensive manner. Demonstrates a broad knowledge of the rules of the game. Has a moderate number of unforced errors per game. Solid understanding of stacking and when and how it could be used in match play. Beginning to identify opponent's weaknesses and attempts to formulate game plan to attack weaknesses. Beginning to seek out more competitive play.

self-rating score	self-rating guideline
4.5	**FOREHAND:** High level of consistency. Uses pace and depth to generate opponents' error or set up next shot. **BACKHAND:** Can effectively direct the ball with varying depth and paces with good consistency. **SERVE/RETURN:** Serves with power, accuracy, and depth and can also vary the speed and spin of the serve. **DINK:** Ability to place ball with high success at changing shot types while playing both consistently and with offensive intent. Recognizes and attempts to hit attackable dinks. **3RD SHOT:** Consistently executes effective 3rd shot strategies that are not easily returned for advantage. Able to intentionally and consistently place the ball. **VOLLEY:** Able to block hard volleys directed at them and can consistently drop them into the NVZ. Comfortable hitting swinging volleys. Hits overhead shots consistently, often as putaways. **STRATEGY:** Has good footwork and moves laterally, backward, and forward well. Uses weight transfer for more efficient footwork. Able to change direction with ease. Very comfortable playing at the Non-Volley Zone. Communicates and moves well with partner — easily "stacks" court positions. Understands strategy and can adjust style of play and game plan according to the opponent's strengths and weaknesses and court position. Limited number of unforced errors.

self-rating score	self-rating guideline
5.0	**FOREHAND/BACKHAND/SERVE/RETURN:** Hits all shot types at a high level of ability from both the forehand and backhand sides including: touch, spin, and pace with control to set up offensive situations. Has developed good touch from all court positions. Has developed a very high level of variety, depth, and pace of serves. **DINK:** Mastered the dink and drop shots. Ability to move opponents with shot placements. Exhibits patience during rallies with the ability to create an opportunity to attack utilizing the dink. Increased ability to change the pace of dinks strategically. **3RD SHOT:** Mastered the 3rd shot choices and strategies to create opportunities for winning points. Able to drop and drive ball from both the forehand and backhand side with high level of consistency. **VOLLEY:** Able to block hard volleys directed at them and consistently drop them into the NVZ. Places overheads with ease for winners. Able to volley shots toward opponents feet consistently. Comfortable with swinging volley in both initiating and ability to attack back or neutralize return. **STRATEGY:** Mastered pickleball strategies and can vary strategies and styles of play in competitive or tournament matches. Is successful at turning defensive shots into offensive shots. Has efficient footwork and effective use of weight transfer for improved quickness on the court. Easily and quickly adjusts style of play and game plan according to the opponent's strengths and weaknesses and court position. Rarely makes unforced errors.

self-rating score	self-rating guideline
5.5+	This player is a top caliber player. Performance and tournament wins speak for this player's ability to consistently perform at a high level.

UTPR PLAYER TOURNAMENT RATINGS SUMMARY

The following tables are from **usapickleball.org**

pickleballtournaments.com ratings
Is a manual rating that is entered into a player's pickleballtournaments.com profile
Is managed and updated by the player
Is the player's opinion of his/her own skill set and is the rating frequently used for non-sanctioned events
Will continue to exist for players that are not members of the USAPA and never play a sanctioned event

USAPA Tournament Player Rating (UTPR)
Is the calculated player rating, based on tournament win/loss results
Have both a 4-digit calculated rating and a rounded down 2-digit skill level
Is the official USA Pickleball rating for sanctioned tournament play. Players may have a doubles, mixed doubles and a singles rating (one for each type of event they participate in)
Is the official rating used to register for USA Pickleball sanctioned tournaments

PLAY-BY-PLAY EXAMPLES OF SCORING IN DOUBLES

Sample scenario

Take a look at the tables below that shows the different aspects of a doubles pickleball game.

Note: We are calling one team AB and the other team CD. **Team AB** starts the game as the **serving team**. **Team CD** is the **receiving team**.

Remember: The **first game of a match** starts begins at **0-0-2**. The team that is serving first only gets **one service turn** before the serve goes to the other team. This means that if the serving team **wins** the first rally, they score a point, and the score becomes 1-0. If the serving team **loses** the first rally, then the serve goes to the other team and the score remains 0-0.

Let's look at some scenarios.

"0" is the serving team's score; "0" is the receiving team's score; the "2" represents that the serving team has only one chance to serve (the opening score exception).

Scenario	Server	Rally winner	Outcome
1. **Team AB** wins the toss and serves. The score is **0-0-2**. They **win** the rally.	The **server (B)** from **Team AB**, serving from the right service court. The server needs to loudly call out the score – 0-0-2 – before serving.	**Team AB**	**Team AB** scores a point, the score is now 1-0-2, and the **server (B)** from **Team AB** continues to serve from the left service court. The server needs to loudly call out the score – 1-0-2 – before serving.
If **Team AB** wins the rally after Scenario 1 above, then **Team AB** scores another point, making the score 2-0-2. The **server (B)** from **Team AB** would then serve again from the right service court. The serving team continues to serve and alternate servers as long as they keep winning the rallies and scoring points.			
2. **Team AB** wins the toss and serves. The score is **0-0-2**. They **lose** the rally.	The **server (B)** from **Team AB**, serving from the right service court. The server needs to loudly call out the score – 0-0-2 – before serving.	**Team CD**	No point is scored, the score is now 0-0-1. **Team CD** now serves. After this first side out, each side has two service turns.

Scenario 1:

- **Server (B)** from **Team AB** is **Ben**. He announces or calls out the score – **0-0-2** – before serving. Ben serves the ball to **Player C (Chris)**, the serve is good, and a rally begins. A rally continues but **Player D (David)** hits the ball out of bounds – that's a point for the serving team (**AB**).
- **Player B (Ben)** continues to serve, but Ben and **Player A (Alex)** switch sides. So, Ben serves again but this time from the left side of the court and to **Player D (David)**. Before he serves, Ben calls out the score **1-0-2**.

Scenario 2:

- **Server** (**B**) from **Team AB** is **Ben**. He announces or calls out the score **0-0-2** before serving. Ben serves the ball to **Player C** (**Chris**), the serve is good, and a rally begins. The rally continues. One of the players from **Team AB** hits the ball out of bounds. No point is scored. **After this first side out**, each side has two service turns. **Team CD** now serves.

If Scenario 2 occurs, what could happen next?

Scenario	Server	Rally winner	Outcome
The score is now 0-0-1. (Scenario 2) 3. **Team CD** serves and wins the rally.	**Player C** from **Team CD**, serving from their right service court. Server C needs to loudly call out the score – 0-0-1 – before serving.	Team CD	**Team CD** scores a point, the score is now 1-0-1, and **Server 1 (C)** from **Team CD** continues to serve from their left service court. Server 1 needs to loudly call out the score – 1-0-1 – before serving.

If **Server 1** from **Team CD** wins the rally after Scenario 3 above, then **Team CD** scores another point, making the score 2-0-1. **Server 1** from **Team CD** would then serve again from the right service court. The serving team continues to serve and alternate servers as long as they keep winning the rallies and scoring points. Only the serving team can score points.

Scenario	Server	Rally winner	Outcome
The score is now 0-0-1. (Scenario 2) 4. **Team CD** serves but loses the rally.	**Server 1 (C)** from **Team CD**, serving from their right service court. Server 1 needs to loudly call out the score – 0-0-1 – before serving.	Team AB	No point is scored. However, now **Server 2** from **Team CD (Player D)** has a turn at serving. If Team CD lose this point, the serve goes back to Team AB. Server 2 needs to loudly call out the score – 0-0-2 – before serving.

Scenario 3:

- The current score is 0-0-1 and Team CD is now serving.
- **Server 1** (**C**) from **Team CD** is **Chris**. She announces the score – 0-0-1 – before serving. Chris serves the ball from the right hand side to **Player B** (**Ben**), the serve is good, and a rally begins. The rally continues. **Player A** (**Alex**) hits the ball out of bounds – that's a point for the serving team (**CD**).
- **Player C** (**Chris**) continues to serve, but Chris and **Player D** (**David**) switch sides. So, Chris serves again but this time from the left side of the court and to **Player A** (**Alex**). Before she serves, Chris calls out the score **1-0-1**.

Scenario 4:

- The current score is 0-0-1 and Team CD is now serving.
- **Server 1** (**C**) from **Team CD** is **Chris**. She announces out the score **0-0-1** before serving. Chris serves the ball to **Player A** (**Alex**) and a rally begins. The rally continues. **Player D** (**David**) hits the ball out of bounds. No point is scored but the serve goes to **Server 2** (**D**) from **Team CD** (**David**).
- **Server 2** (**D**) (**David**) calls out the score – **0-0-2** – before serving from the right side to **Player B** (**Ben**).

Remember, at the start of the game, only one player gets to serve from the serving team (the team that has won the toss). If a point is scored, the server switches sides with their partner and serves again. When they lose a rally (commit a fault) and the serving switches to the other team, both players in each team then get to serve, one after the other. A player loses their serve when their team loses a rally. A point can only be scored by the serving team.

DRILLS TO HONE YOUR SKILLS: PERFECTING YOUR PERFORMANCE

Throughout this book, you have seen examples of different types of **drills**.

As you will recall, a **pickleball drill** is an exercise designed to isolate and work on a particular skill or set of skills that a player desires to improve. Drills offer players many benefits, including improved technique, cardiovascular fitness, strength, and muscle memory gains. By committing skills to muscle memory through drilling, players can react and respond instinctively while using their mental skills to focus on strategy on the court .

CORE PICKLEBALL SKILLS

Before diving into specific pickleball stroke skills and how to drill them, it's important to start by identifying the basic and broader athletic skills that are needed as a foundation to play well in pickleball and need to be present every time you step out to drill. Three important core pickleball skills are having an **athletic ready stance**, **balance** and **footwork**.

The **athletic ready stance** is essential in pickleball. It means you're in a position ready to move in any direction, have your paddle ready to return a shot, and are prepared to play the ball off of a bounce or in the air.

- **Sample drill**: **Lateral shuffle and stop**
  This drill improves your ability to quickly get into an athletic ready stance. Start at one sideline of the pickleball court. Shuffle laterally to the other sideline and abruptly stop, ensuring you are in an athletic ready stance. Repeat this back and forth, emphasizing quick, smooth movement, and an abrupt stop into a solid athletic ready stance.

Maintaining **balance** during play is crucial for controlled, accurate shots.

- **Sample drill**: **Single-leg balance with paddle work**
  To perform this drill, stand on one leg while maintaining balance. While balanced on one leg, pass your pickleball paddle around your body in various directions to mimic the diverse range of motion required during a game. After a set time or number of passes, switch to balance on the other leg.

Effective **footwork** can make a big difference in your ability to reach balls and return them accurately and powerfully.

Sample drill: Pickleball ladder drills

Using a ladder or a series of lines on the ground, you can practice various footwork patterns. Two footwork drills you might use include:

- **Two feet in each square**: Begin at one end of the ladder. Moving sideways, place both feet in the first square, then both feet in the second square, and so on, until you reach the end of the ladder. Try to move as quickly as you can while maintaining control.

- **In-in-out-out**: Starting from the side of the ladder, step with your lead foot into the first square, followed by your other foot. Then step out with your lead foot followed by your other foot. Repeat this pattern down the entire length of the ladder.

Athletic ready stance, balance, and footwork are essential skills for being able to move quickly and efficiently on the court. For example, imagine you're playing a doubles match and your opponent hits a shot to the far corner of the court. If you're in an athletic ready stance with your weight evenly distributed over both feet, you'll be able to quickly push off and move towards the ball. If your center of gravity is lower to the ground with your knees bent and your paddle up and ready, you'll be able to maintain balance as you move and be ready to hit the ball when you get there. Even if the ball isn't coming close to you, it's important to maintain good form and be ready to move at all times.

Drills can help improve these skills by putting you into a repeatedly stressed, constantly moving position that you simply cannot achieve during a game. For example, a drill that involves repeatedly hitting the ball between two players on either side of the net is far more taxing than playing a point during a game. This type of drill can help improve your athletic ready stance, balance, and footwork by forcing you to maintain good form while constantly moving and hitting the ball.

TYPES OF DRILLS – SOLO DRILLS AND DOUBLES DRILLS

Solo drills are technical and repeated exercises that can be done by a player alone to improve their skills and technique. These types of drills can help a player develop their footwork, agility, reaction time, hand-eye coordination, ball control, and serve accuracy. Solo drills can be done on a pickleball court or on a practice wall.

Doubles drills, on the other hand, are designed to be done with a partner. These types of drills can help players improve their doubles game by working on skills such as serve/return, 3rd shots, dinks, drives, lobs, resets/blocks, and everything in between. Doubles drills can help players develop their teamwork, communication, and strategy. For example,

1. **Skinny singles or half-court singles**: This drill emulates the strategy and play of doubles, but you have the opportunity to play every shot and work on your skills on every shot. Players take turns serving and returning, and play out points on half of the court.
2. **Cross-court dinks**: In this drill, players stand diagonally across from each other at the Non-Volley Zone line and hit dinks back and forth cross-court .
3. **Forehand and backhand dinks**: In this drill, players stand across from each other at the Non-Volley Zone line and hit dinks back and forth using only their forehand or backhand
4. **Triangle dinks**: In this drill, three players stand at the Non-Volley Zone line forming a triangle. One player hits a dink to one of the other players, who then hits a dink to the third player, who then hits a dink back to the first player.

Finding a **drill partner** can make drilling more fun and competitive. One way to make drilling more enjoyable is to play competitive games during drilling sessions.

SOME OTHER USEFUL DRILLS

- **Wall ball drill**

This drill helps improve your control, accuracy, and reflexes. Stand about 10 feet away from a wall and hit the ball against it, then try to hit it again on the rebound. You can adjust the speed, angle, and placement of your shots to increase the difficulty and simulate different game situations.

- **Serve and return drill**

With a partner, one player serves while the other player returns the serve. The server focuses on serving to different areas of the service box, while the returner works on returning serves to the desired location on the court. After several serves, switch roles. This is a great way to practice both your serve and your return.

- **Dinking drill**

Dinking is an essential skill in pickleball that involves hitting the ball softly over the net to land within the Non-Volley Zone (also known as the kitchen). Practice your dinks by standing at the kitchen line and dinking the ball back and forth with a partner. Aim for consistency and precision, trying to make each shot as difficult as possible for your partner to return.

- **Third shot drop drill**

The third shot drop is a technique that is used to transition from the baseline to the kitchen line. One player starts at the baseline, the other at the kitchen line. The baseline player initiates a rally with a deep shot, and then the kitchen line player returns the ball deep. The baseline player then attempts a third shot drop—a soft shot intended to arc over the net and land in the kitchen. The kitchen player lets the ball bounce once before returning it, and then both players proceed to play out the point.

- **Volley drill**

In this drill, both players stand at the kitchen line and hit volleys back and forth without letting the ball bounce. This drill can help improve your reaction times and your ability to accurately hit volleys.

These drills should help you improve different aspects of your pickleball game, from serves and returns to dinking and volleying.

PICKLEBALL EVENTS AND TOURNAMENTS IN THE USA

There are many pickleball events and tournaments held throughout the year in the USA. Some of the largest pickleball tournaments include:

USA Pickleball National Championships: This is one of the most prestigious tournaments in the U.S. The tournament usually takes place in November, and it brings together the best players from all over the country.

Minto US Open Pickleball Championships: Another highly competitive and prestigious event, the US Open usually happens annually in Naples, Florida. It's one of the largest pickleball events worldwide and attracts a wide array of international talent.

Professional Pickleball Association (PPA) Tour Events: This professional tour hosts several tournaments across the country, often featuring cash prizes and high levels of competition.

Association of Pickleball Professionals (APP) Tour Events: Another professional tour, the APP also runs several high-level tournaments across the United States each year.

Tournament of Champions: Held in Brigham City, Utah, this tournament features pro and senior pro events and is one of the premier tournaments on the pickleball calendar.

IFP Bainbridge Cup: This is an international team competition created by the International Federation of Pickleball (IFP) in 2017 to foster competition among the world's countries. The tournament honors the birthplace of pickleball, Bainbridge Island, Washington, and the venue moves to different locations around the world every year 12. The inaugural IFP Bainbridge Cup took place in 2017 in Madrid, Spain, and was the first intercontinental pickleball team event in the history of the sport

RESOURCES FOR IMPROVING YOUR GAME

As we have seen, pickleball is a fast-growing sport that is enjoyed by people of all ages and skill levels. Whether you are a beginner just starting out or an experienced player looking to take your game to the next level, there are many resources available to help you improve.

In this section, we have compiled a list of **websites**, **YouTube channels** and **blogs** that provide valuable information about the sport of pickleball. These resources offer instructional videos, tips and tricks, and insights from top players and coaches. By accessing these websites, YouTube channels, blogs, and other **social media sites**, you can learn new techniques, strategies, and tactics to help you become a better pickleball player. So, whether you want to improve your serve, work on your footwork, or learn how to play smarter, these resources are a great place to start.

Top websites, YouTube channels, blogs, and other social media sites

USA Pickleball – usapickleball.org

USA Pickleball is the national governing body for the sport of pickleball in the US. It provides players with official rules, tournaments, rankings, and more. Their **website** offers a variety of resources for players, including instructional videos, tips and tricks, and insights from top players and coaches. Additionally, the website has a section called "Master the Basics" which includes videos on how to play pickleball, basics for success, and more. They also offer 5 free bonus videos and a free e-book when you sign up. You can also follow USA Pickleball on **Facebook**, **Instagram**, **TikTok**, **Twitter** and **YouTube**.

pickleball.com

pickleball.com is a **website** that provides information and resources about the sport of pickleball. The website offers a variety of resources for pickleball players, including articles, videos, instructional courses, an online shop, and a community forum.

Pickleball Canada – pickleballcanada.org

The **Pickleball Canada website** is the official online resource for the national governing body of pickleball in Canada. The site provides a wealth of information and resources for players, including details on basic rules, coaching, tournaments, ratings, and officiating. By becoming a member of Pickleball Canada, players can access additional benefits such as eligibility to enter sanctioned tournaments and training for officiating. The organization is dedicated to promoting the growth and development of pickleball throughout Canada.

Pickleball Central – pickleballcentral.com

Pickleballcentral.com is an online platform dedicated to serving the pickleball community. It offers a wide range of resources, including informative articles, instructional videos, and expert advice, to help players improve their skills and knowledge of the game. The website also provides a diverse selection of pickleball equipment and fosters a sense of community through forums, blogs, and user reviews.

Pickleball Coach – pickleballcoach.com

Pickleballcoach.com is a **website** that offers instructional materials for pickleball players, including DVDs and books. The site features resources created by a well-known and respected figure in the pickleball community, **Coach Mo**. One of the top-selling products on the site is a DVD that provides instruction on various topics, including grip, ready position, forehand groundstroke, stances, backhand groundstroke, volley, footwork, serve, return of serve, and more. The site also offers a book that provides a complete guide to playing pickleball. There is also a **YouTube** channel.

Pickleball Kitchen – pickleballkitchen.com

PickleballKitchen.com is a **website**, **podcast**, and **YouTube** channel dedicated to helping players at all levels of their pickleball journey. The website provides information for both beginners and experienced players, including tips, gear reviews, and articles on the history of pickleball.

The website was created by Barrett Kincheloe, a PPR and IPTPA certified instructor, writer, podcaster, and YouTuber with the goal of helping as many people as possible with pickleball. Barrett strongly believes that pickleball can positively impact people's lives.

The website features a variety of content including written articles, podcast episodes, and videos on the Pickleball Kitchen YouTube channel. The content covers a wide range of topics such as tips for improving your serve, keeping your paddle in "Ready Position", improving your dink, or playing the fast game against better players

The Pickler – thepickler.com

Pickler is a pickleball content and media brand that was launched in 2017. Its mission is to promote the sport of pickleball and inspire others to play pickleball. Pickler strives to help pickleball players improve their game and play their best. Whether you're a beginner just starting out or an experienced player looking to take your game to the next level, The Pickler is a comprehensive resource for pickleball players.

thepickler.com is a **website** that offers a wealth of resources for pickleball players looking to improve their game. The website provides instructional videos, tips and tricks, and insights from top players and coaches, all designed to help players learn new techniques, strategies, and tactics. In addition to the instructional content, The Pickler also has a blog section where they share tips and stories about pickleball, as well as a bi-weekly newsletter that provides tips, strategies, stories, and the latest news from the best in the game. You can also follow Pickler on **Facebook**, **Instagram**, **TikTok**, **Twitter** and **YouTube**.

The Pickleball Studio

The **Pickleball Studio** is a popular **YouTube channel** that provides a variety of content related to the sport of pickleball. The channel is run by Chris Olson, who is well-known and respected in the pickleball community . The channel features videos on a range of topics, including paddle reviews, tips and strategies, interviews with players and industry experts, and more. With over 12.5K subscribers and 120 videos, The Pickleball Studio is a great resource for anyone interested in learning more about the sport of pickleball.

Pickleball Pirates

The **Pickleball Pirates** is a **YouTube channel** that features videos of amateur non-pro pickleball players on their quest to reach a 5.0 skill level. The channel has over 11.9K subscribers and features over 2K videos. The content on the channel includes instructional videos, tips, and highlights of recreational play.

Pickleball Portal – pickleballportal.com

Pickleballportal.com is a **website** dedicated to providing information and resources related to the sport of pickleball. The site covers everything from the history of the game to gear reviews, tips, and strategies for players of all skill levels. The site also features a Pickleball FAQ section with answers to dozens of common questions about the game. Whether you are new to the sport or an experienced player, pickleballportal.com is a great resource for all things pickleball.

PPA Tour YouTube Channel – www.youtube.com/c/PPAtour

The **PPA Tour YouTube channel** is the official channel of the Carvana Professional Pickleball Association (PPA), which is home to some of the best professional pickleball players. The channel has over 44.8K subscribers and features 968 videos. The channel provides a great way for fans to keep up with the latest action from PPA Tour tournaments across the country.

Pickleball University – pickleballuniversity.com

PickleballUniversity.com is a **website** that exists to educate and entertain beginning and experienced players alike with tips, gear reviews, and videos around one of the world's fastest-growing sports. The website provides information for players of all skill levels to help them improve their game and learn more about the sport of pickleball.

Pickleheads – pickleheads.com

Pickleheads.com is a **website** that helps players discover local pickleball courts and games. The website has a comprehensive list of indoor and outdoor pickleball courts in the US and Canada, with over 13,000 places to play. Users can filter courts by court type, surface, amenities, lighting, and more. Pickleheads also allows users to join a community of pickleball players, discover local games, and recruit nearby players. In addition to helping players find courts and games, Pickleheads also offers a free scheduling tool for pickleball organizers. The website also includes a blog with articles on how to play pickleball, gear reviews, and other topics related to the sport.

GLOSSARY: KEY PICKLEBALL TERMS EXPLAINED

ace: An ace in pickleball refers to a serve that lands in the opponent's court untouched, resulting in an immediate point for the serving team.

angle selection: In pickleball, 'angle selection' refers to choosing the best direction to hit the ball during a rally. It involves assessing the court and opponents to determine the most effective angle for your shot. The goal is to strategically place the ball in areas that make it difficult for your opponent to return.

anticipation: Anticipation refers to the ability to predict and foresee your opponent's shots or intentions before they are executed. It involves reading cues from your opponent's body language, positioning, and shot selection patterns to anticipate the direction, pace, and type of shot they are likely to play.

approach shot or approach stroke: A shot played while moving toward the net, typically used to set up an offensive opportunity.

Around the Post (ATP): A specialty shot in pickleball where you hit the ball under the top of the net and around the net post1. This is a legal shot where the player hits the ball around the post and into their opponent's court without crossing into their half of the court.

Association of Pickleball Professionals (APP): A professional organization dedicated to promoting and advancing the sport of pickleball.

athletic stance: Refers to the balanced and ready position adopted by a player in preparation for engaging in a physical activity or sport. In pickleball, the athletic stance is the foundational position that allows players to react quickly, maintain stability, and generate power and agility. It involves standing with feet shoulder-width apart, knees slightly bent, weight evenly distributed on both feet, and the body centered and aligned.

attack: In pickleball, an attack refers to a forceful offensive shot made with the intention of putting pressure on the opponent and gaining an advantage in the rally. It typically involves hitting the ball with power and accuracy to create difficulty for the opponent in returning the shot.

attackable ball: An attackable ball in pickleball refers to a shot or serve that is positioned in a way that allows the receiving player to aggressively and effectively attack the ball. It is a favorable opportunity for the receiving player to make an offensive shot, typically with the goal of gaining control of the rally or scoring a point.

backcourt: This refers to the area of the court located towards the back or rear end of the playing area. It is the section of the court that is farther away from the net. Players typically occupy the backcourt when defending against their opponents' shots and preparing for their own offensive plays.

backhand: A shot executed with the non-dominant hand on the side of the body opposite to the hand holding the paddle. It is a stroke where the player strikes the ball using the backside or the top side of the paddle, depending on the technique employed.

backspin: A spin applied to the ball in which it rotates backward, causing it to slow down, drop quickly, and potentially bounce backward after landing.

backswing: The motion of the paddle and arm swinging backward before striking the ball, generating power and momentum for the shot.

banger: A player known for hitting powerful shots with significant speed and force, often aiming to overwhelm opponents with aggressive play.

baseline: The boundary line at the back of the pickleball court, marking the farthest point from the net.

behind the back shot: A shot played by hitting the ball while reaching behind the back, showcasing exceptional skill and coordination.

bert: A "Bert" is an advanced shot in pickleball that is similar to an "Erne" shot, but it is executed on your partner's side of the court. It involves a player crossing the court into their partner's half to perform a maneuver that avoids the Non-Volley Zone and slams the ball right at the net at a sharp angle down to the opponents' feet.

block/block volley: A defensive shot where the player positions their paddle in front of an incoming ball to stop or redirect it, typically executed near the net.

body shot: A shot aimed directly at the opponent's body, designed to limit their ability to return the ball effectively.

bye: In a tournament or competition, a bye refers to a situation where a player or team advances to the next round without having to play a match, typically due to an odd number of participants or a predetermined arrangement.

calling the score: In pickleball, the score is called before each serve. The proper sequence for calling the score is: server score, receiver score, and for doubles only, the server number one or two. To start a pickleball match, the score will be called zero, zero, two. This means that as soon as the serving team commits a fault, the other team gets to serve.

cardiovascular exercises: Activities that elevate the heart rate, increase blood circulation, and warm up the entire body.

carry: This refers to an illegal shot where the player holds or carries the ball on the paddle for too long instead of striking it cleanly. This is against the rules and results in a fault, leading to the loss of the rally and a point for the opposing team. The ball should be struck cleanly and without excessive contact or prolonged holding on the paddle.

centerline: The centerline in pickleball is the line that divides the court into two equal halves, separating the left and right sides of the court.

closed paddle face: This refers to the angle of the paddle when it makes contact with the ball. When the paddle face is closed, it is angled towards the ground, which can cause the ball to be hit into the net or to have a lower trajectory.

composite: Refers to pickleball paddle construction using a combination of materials such as graphite, fiberglass, or other composites, offering enhanced performance characteristics such as durability, power, and control.

conditioning: This refers to the physical preparation and training necessary to enhance overall fitness, strength, endurance, and agility.

continental grip: A grip style where the hand is positioned in such a way that the knuckles align diagonally across the paddle handle, allowing for versatility in executing various shots with ease.

controlled placement This refers to the intentional and strategic placement of your defensive shots. It involves hitting the ball with precision and accuracy to specific areas of the court that make it difficult for your opponents to launch effective attacks.

cool down: Cool down refers to the period of reduced intensity following exercise or physical activity, typically performed at the end of a workout. It involves engaging in gentle exercises or activities to gradually lower the heart rate, regulate breathing, and allow the body to return to its pre-exercise state. The purpose of a cool down is to promote recovery, prevent muscle soreness, and facilitate the transition from exercise back to a resting state.

court coverage: Court coverage is the ability to move and position oneself on the pickleball court to effectively respond to shots from opponents. It involves anticipating and reaching incoming shots, maintaining balance, and reacting quickly.

crossover step: A footwork technique in pickleball that involves crossing one foot over the other while moving in a lateral or diagonal direction. It is commonly used to quickly change direction and cover ground on the court. When executing the crossover step, the player steps one foot over the other in a crossing motion, allowing for a smooth transition and efficient movement.

cross step: A footwork technique where a player steps one foot across the front of the other foot, enabling efficient movement and balance while transitioning to different areas of the court.

crosscourt: Refers to a shot that is hit diagonally from one side of the court to the other, landing in the opposite service court

cross-court dink: Refers to a soft shot played diagonally across the net, aimed at landing in the opponent's Non-Volley Zone.

cutthroat pickleball: A variation of the game that involves three players instead of the traditional two.

dead ball: Refers to a ball that is no longer in play due to any action that stops play, such as a fault or a hinder. When a fault occurs, the ball is declared dead, and the rally ends.

dedicated court: This is a court that is specifically designed and used only for playing pickleball. It can be an indoor or outdoor court, and it is marked with the appropriate lines and has a net set up at the correct height for pickleball play.

deep serve: A strategic serve that lands closer to the back boundary line of the receiving side.

defensive shots: In pickleball are shots that are used to defend against an opponent's attack and to buy time for the player to recover and get back into position. Some examples of defensive shots include the lob, which is hit high and deep into the opponent's court to give the player time to recover, and the block shot, which is used to block power and quick shots from the opponent.

defensive slices: A shot that is hit with underspin, causing the ball to have a low trajectory and bounce low, making it difficult for the opponent to attack. It can be used as a defensive shot to buy time for the player to recover and get back into position.

dig: A defensive shot used to return a hard-hit ball that is close to the ground. The player will often have to bend low and reach out with their paddle to make contact with the ball, using a quick upward motion to lift the ball back over the net. It is a difficult shot that requires quick reflexes and good hand-eye coordination.

dink: A soft and controlled shot played with finesse and precision, usually executed close to the net, aiming to place the ball in the opponent's Non-Volley Zone and disrupt their positioning.

dink volley: A soft shot that is hit out of the air before the ball bounces, with the intention of placing the ball into the opponent's Non-Volley Zone (also known as the kitchen). It is a controlled shot that requires touch and finesse, and is used to neutralize fast playing and rallying shots from the baselines

dinking: Dinking in pickleball is a soft shot hit into the opponent's Non-Volley Zone to neutralize fast shots and move the game closer to the net. It forces the opponent to let the ball bounce before returning it.

double bounce rule: The double bounce refers to the rule that mandates the ball must bounce once on each side of the net at the start of the rally, ensuring fair play and allowing for proper positioning before players engage in volleys.

double hit: A double hit in pickleball occurs when a player hits the ball twice consecutively without the ball touching any other surface or player in between. It is generally considered an illegal shot, as per the rules of the game. A double hit is considered a fault and results in a point being awarded to the opposing team. Players are allowed to hit the ball only once during their shot execution, ensuring fair play and maintaining the integrity of the game.

doubles: A game format in pickleball where two players form a team on each side of the net, competing against another doubles team.

doubles partner: The teammate or partner with whom a player teams up to compete in doubles matches, working together to strategize and cover the court.

drills: Drills in pickleball refer to structured practice exercises designed to improve specific aspects of a player's game. They involve repetitive and focused repetitions of specific movements, shots, strategies, or skills, aiming to enhance technique, footwork, decision-making, and overall performance on the court.

drive: A forceful and offensive shot hit with power and speed, typically aimed to pass opponents and score points.

drop-in play: In pickleball, this refers to an informal setting where players can show up to the courts and join a game without prior scheduling or registration. It is a welcoming and inclusive environment where players of all skill levels, ages, and backgrounds can come together to play the game.

drop serve: A drop serve in pickleball is an alternative serving technique that was introduced in 2021 and made permanent. It involves dropping the ball from the non-dominant hand, letting it bounce once, and then hitting it with the paddle. It can provide more control and accuracy for the server.

drop shot: A soft and intentionally placed shot that is played with finesse and minimal power, aiming to land the ball close to the net and make it difficult for the opponent to return.

drop volley: A volley executed with a gentle touch and control, resulting in a soft shot close to the net, often used to place the ball strategically and disrupt the opponent's positioning.

DUPR: DUPR stands for Dynamic Universal Pickleball Rating. It is the most accurate and only global rating system in pickleball. All players, regardless of their age, gender, location, or skill, are rated on the same scale between 2.000-8.000 based on their match results. DUPR is free to register, and anyone can have a rating.

dynamic stretches: Active stretching exercises that involve moving parts of your body through a full range of motion. These stretches are performed in a controlled and deliberate manner, mimicking the movements used in pickleball.

eastern grip: The eastern grip is a common pickleball grip where the hand is positioned slightly to the right side of the paddle (for right-handed players), with the index knuckle on the edge of the paddle and the remaining fingers wrapped around the handle. It provides balance and versatility for different shots.

edge guard: An edge guard refers to a protective strip or edge tape applied to the paddle face to prevent damage or wear along the paddle's edges.

edgeless paddle: An edgeless paddle is a type of paddle design without a distinct edge or rim, providing a larger paddle face and eliminating the possibility of hitting the ball with the edge.

Elo rating system: The Elo rating system is a method for calculating the relative skill levels of players in zero-sum games. It takes into account factors such as the player's skill level and the result of the match to calculate a player's rating, which increases or decreases depending on the outcome of games between rated players.

erne: Named after Erne Perry, this is an advanced shot in pickleball where you hit the ball either in the air as you are jumping around the Non-Volley Zone (the kitchen) or after you run around or through the kitchen and re-establish your feet out of bounds, just to the side of the kitchen In either case, it is on your side of the pickleball court.

etiquette: A set of unwritten rules that govern social behavior, ensuring respect, consideration, and fairness among individuals.

even court: This refers to the right side of the court when facing the net. The server stands on the even court when their score is even. It also refers to a scenario in pickleball where both teams have an equal score, such as 0-0, 2-2, or any even number of points.

face of the paddle: The face of the paddle refers to the surface area of the pickleball paddle that makes contact with the ball during play.

fair play: This refers to the adherence to the rules and spirit of the game, ensuring equal opportunities, unbiased judgment, and honorable conduct.

fault: A fault is a violation or an error that results in the loss of a rally, often occurring when a serve does not land in the correct service box, the ball is hit out-of-bounds, or a rule is broken.

finesse: Finesse refers to the skillful and delicate control of shots, emphasizing touch, placement, and precision rather than power or force. It involves the ability to manipulate the ball with subtle and controlled movements, often using softer shots that require finesse rather than sheer strength.

first server: The first server refers to the player who initiates the serving at the beginning of a game or after a side out. The first server has the responsibility to serve the ball into the diagonal service court of the opposing team.

first-server band: In pickleball doubles, a first server band is a form of identification worn by the player who serves first for their team. It is typically a wristband or other visible marker that helps players keep track of who served first and avoid confusion during the game.

follow through: The continuation of the paddle swing motion after making contact with the ball, which ensures control, power, and accuracy in executing shots.

foot fault: In pickleball, a foot fault can occur in two ways. One is when a player volleys the ball inside the kitchen (Non-Volley Zone). If a player passes the Non-Volley Zone line and stands in the kitchen, they must let the ball bounce once before hitting it. Another way is when the serving player's foot crosses over the baseline during a serve. The serve must be performed behind the baseline.

forehand: A forehand shot is one where the player strikes the ball with the paddle on the dominant hand's side of the body (right side for right-handed players, left side for left-handed players).

game: A game refers to the segment of play in pickleball where players compete to reach a specific number of points, usually 11 or 15, to win the game.

game point: In pickleball, a game point is the point that, if won by the serving team, would result in them winning the game. Most games in pickleball are played to 11 points (win by 2), although some pickleball games in tournament settings may be played to 15 points (win by 2) or 21 points (win by 2)

gender doubles: Gender doubles refers to a doubles game format in which teams consist of players of the same gender, such as all-male or all-female teams.

Global Pickleball Rankings (GPR): This is a ranking system based on ranking points. The value of the ranking points is defined by the tournament tier and skill levels.

good sportsmanship: This refers to the conduct, attitude, and behavior of players, characterized by integrity, respect, and fairness towards opponents, officials, and the game itself. It embodies the spirit of competition while maintaining a sense of fairness, ethical behavior, and respect for the rules.

graphite: Graphite is a lightweight and durable material commonly used in the construction of pickleball paddles, known for its excellent strength-to-weight ratio and responsiveness.

grip: A grip refers to how a player holds the paddle, with different grip styles including the Continental grip, Eastern grip, Western grip, and variations in between.

grip pressure: The amount of force or tightness with which a player holds the pickleball paddle during gameplay.

grip tape: Adhesive tapes wrapped around the handle of a pickleball paddle to enhance grip and prevent slipping.

groundstroke: A groundstroke is a shot played after the ball has bounced, where the player hits the ball after it has made contact with the court surface, typically executed from the backcourt to keep the ball in play.

half court: Half court in pickleball refers to playing on only one side of the net, usually in practice or recreational settings, where players take turns hitting shots to each other without crossing the net.

half stack: In pickleball, half stack refers to a serving team formation where one player stands at the Non-Volley Zone line and the other player positions slightly behind and towards the middle of the court.

half-volley: A half-volley is a shot where the player hits the ball immediately after it bounces off the ground, requiring precise timing and skill to make contact with the ball just as it rises from the surface.

handle: The handle of a pickleball paddle refers to the part of the paddle grip that a player holds onto during play, providing control and stability.

hydration break: A hydration break is a brief pause during a game or match to allow players to hydrate and replenish fluids, ensuring their well-being and performance during play.

IFP (International Federation of Pickleball): The International Federation of Pickleball (IFP) is the global governing body for the sport of pickleball. It is responsible for overseeing and promoting the development of pickleball worldwide, establishing and enforcing the official rules of the game, organizing international competitions and events, and fostering the growth and recognition of pickleball as a sport on a global scale. The IFP plays a crucial role in coordinating and unifying pickleball efforts across different countries, supporting the development of national pickleball organizations, and ensuring fair and consistent standards for the game. Through its initiatives and partnerships, the IFP strives to enhance the accessibility, inclusivity, and professionalism of pickleball, contributing to the global expansion and recognition of the sport.

injury prevention: This refers to the strategies and practices implemented to minimize the risk of injuries during gameplay. It involves taking proactive measures to protect your body and maintain physical well-being.

inside foot: This refers to the foot closer to the centerline when hitting a shot. It helps with balance, power, and shot execution. By positioning the inside foot correctly, players can generate more power and control in their shots. It is an essential aspect of footwork and technique in pickleball

kitchen: The kitchen, also known as the Non-Volley Zone, is the area on each side of the net that extends 7 feet back from the net. Players are not allowed to step into this zone and hit volleys unless the ball has bounced in this area.

kitchen fault/violation: A kitchen fault or violation occurs when a player steps into the kitchen or hits a volley while standing inside the Non-Volley Zone, resulting in the loss of a rally or point.

kitchen line: The kitchen line refers to the boundary line that marks the front edge of the Non-Volley Zone or kitchen area on each side of the net.

league: A pickleball league is an organized competition where players or teams participate in a series of matches against other players or teams within the league, often spanning multiple weeks or months.

left/odd service box: The left service box, also known as the odd service box, is the service box on the left-hand side of the court as viewed from the serving team's perspective. It is called the odd service box because it is used when the server's score is odd. In doubles play, the server stands in the right service box if their score is even and in the left service box if their score is odd. The server must serve diagonally to the receiver in the opposite service box on the other side of the net.

line call: A line call in pickleball refers to the judgment made by a player or referee to determine whether a shot or ball landed inside or outside the court boundaries. It involves determining whether the ball touched any part of the line that marks the boundary of the court. Line calls are crucial in determining the outcome of a point and are typically made based on the player's or referee's visual observation of where the ball landed in relation to the court lines.

line judge: A line judge is an official or player assigned to observe specific lines on the court during a match and make line calls to determine whether shots or balls landed in or out.

lob: A lob is a high-arching shot played with the intention of sending the ball over the opponent's head and deep into their backcourt, often used as a defensive or strategic play.

lob volley: A lob volley in pickleball refers to a shot played in the air without allowing the ball to bounce, with a high trajectory aimed at sending the ball over the opponent's head and deep into their backcourt.

lobber: A lobber is a player who frequently uses lobs as a primary strategy in their game, relying on high shots to disrupt opponents' positioning and create opportunities for offensive plays.

match point: Match point refers to the crucial final point needed to win a match, often creating a decisive and tense moment in the game.

midcourt: The midcourt is the central area of the pickleball court, located between the Non-Volley Zone and the baseline, serving as a transition area where players position themselves for shots from both the backcourt and the Non-Volley Zone.

mixed doubles: Mixed doubles is a game format in pickleball where a team consists of one male and one female player, promoting gender diversity and allowing for unique dynamics in the game.

moisture-wicking fabrics: Moisture-wicking fabrics are materials that pull moisture away from the skin, allowing it to evaporate more easily. These fabrics keep the wearer dry and comfortable during physical activities by reducing sweat buildup and the risk of chafing.

moon ball serve: The moon ball serve is a type of serve in pickleball where the server hits the ball high and soft, so that it lands deep in the opponent's court near the baseline.

multiuse court: A multiuse court is a pickleball court that is designed and marked to accommodate multiple sports or activities, offering flexibility for various sports to be played on the same court.

muscle memory: The ability of your muscles to remember and repeat specific movements without conscious thought.

Nasty Nelson: Nasty Nelson is a slang term used to describe a particularly challenging or difficult shot or serve in pickleball, often characterized by its unpredictable trajectory or speed.

neutral flat shots: Shots that are hit with a flat paddle face and minimal spin. These shots are typically played with moderate speed and are aimed to keep the ball low and fast, allowing the player to maintain control of the point and keep the opponent on the defensive. Neutral flat shots are versatile and can be used both offensively and defensively, depending on the situation in the game.

nice get: "Nice get" is an expression used to acknowledge and compliment a player who successfully retrieves a difficult or hard-to-reach shot.

nice rally: "Nice rally" is an expression used to acknowledge and appreciate an exciting and well-played exchange of shots between players during a rally.

nomex: Nomex is used in the construction of some pickleball paddles. It is used as a core material, which is laid between the two faces of the paddle, usually in a honeycomb pattern. This type of core begins as a cardboard-like material and is then dipped in resin to create an extremely durable material.

Non-Volley line: The Non-Volley line, also known as the kitchen line, is the boundary line that marks the front edge of the Non-Volley Zone on each side of the net. Players are not allowed to hit volleys while standing in this zone.

Non-Volley Zone (NVZ or the kitchen): The Non-Volley Zone, also known as the NVZ or the kitchen, is the area on each side of the net that extends 7 feet back from the net. Players are not allowed to hit volleys (shots in the air without the ball bouncing) while standing inside this zone.

Non-Volley Zone violation: A Non-Volley Zone violation in pickleball occurs when a player steps into the Non-Volley Zone (also known as "the kitchen") and volleys the ball (hits it out of the air before it bounces). The Non-Volley Zone is a 7-foot area on either side of the net where players are not allowed to volley the ball. If a player steps into the Non-Volley Zone and volleys the ball, it is considered a fault and results in a point for the opposing team.

Non-Volley Zone fault/violation: A Non-Volley Zone fault or violation occurs when a player hits a volley (shot in the air without the ball bouncing) while standing inside the Non-Volley Zone, resulting in the loss of a rally or point.

no man's land: No man's land refers to the area on the pickleball court between the Non-Volley Zone and the baseline. It is a strategic term used to describe a position where players may find themselves vulnerable, as they are not in an ideal position to execute offensive shots or defensive returns.

odd court: This refers to the left side of the court when facing the net. The server stands on the odd court when their score is odd.

offensive shots: Offensive shots in pickleball refer to aggressive and attacking shots that are aimed at putting pressure on the opponent and winning points.

offensive topspins: Shots that involve imparting topspin on the ball, causing it to rotate forward as it travels over the net. These shots are executed with power and aggressiveness, aiming to create speed and depth in the shot, making it difficult for the opponent to handle and enabling the player to take control of the point.

one-handed backhand A one-handed backhand refers to a backhand shot where the player uses only one hand to strike the ball. Unlike the two-handed backhand, which involves using both hands on the paddle, the one-handed backhand relies on the player's dominant hand to execute the shot.

open paddle face: Open paddle face refers to the position of the paddle face where it is angled more away from the net, resulting in a shot with greater height and less spin, often used for defensive or defensive-like shots.

out ball: Refers to a shot or serve that lands outside the designated boundaries of the court, resulting in the point being awarded to the opposing team. When a ball is deemed out, it means it did not make contact with the playable area, such as the lines or the surface within the court boundaries.

outside foot: The outside foot refers to the foot farthest from the centerline of the court, typically used as a reference point for footwork and positioning during pickleball play.

overgrip: Thin, padded wraps placed over the handle of a pickleball paddle for added cushioning and grip.

overhead: Overhead refers to a shot or stroke played above the player's head, typically executed with the paddle swinging downward and generating power from above.

overhead smash: An overhead smash, also known as a smash or overhead shot, is a forceful and aggressive shot played from above the player's head with the intention of hitting the ball down with power and velocity.

paddle: A paddle in pickleball is a solid, rectangular-shaped racket used to hit the ball. It typically consists of a handle and a larger face made of materials such as graphite, composite, or wood.

paddle contact: Paddle contact in pickleball refers to the act of striking the ball with the pickleball paddle, using proper technique and control to direct the ball.

paddle covers: Protective cases or sleeves designed to cover and safeguard pickleball paddles when not in use, providing protection against dust, scratches, and other potential damage.

paddle edge guards: Protective attachments or strips applied to the edges of pickleball paddles to prevent damage from accidental impacts, collisions, or scrapes during gameplay. They serve as a cushion and barrier, shielding the paddle's edges and prolonging its lifespan.

paddle face: The paddle face refers to the surface area of the pickleball paddle that makes contact with the ball during play.

paddle tap: A paddle tap is a gentle and controlled shot where the player lightly taps the ball with the paddle, typically used for dinking or placing the ball precisely over the net.

permanent object: In pickleball, a permanent object refers to any fixed structure or obstacle that is present within the boundaries of the pickleball court. This can include items such as posts, fences, or other immovable structures. These permanent objects are considered to be in play during the game, meaning that if the ball touches or interacts with them, it is still considered a valid shot.

pickler: A pickler refers to an enthusiastic player or fan of pickleball, someone who enjoys and actively participates in the sport.

pickleballs: Pickleballs are the lightweight, perforated plastic balls used in pickleball play. They have a unique design with holes that reduce air resistance and provide a slower speed compared to traditional tennis balls.

pickleball court: A pickleball court is a playing surface where the game of pickleball is played. It is similar to a badminton court in size and layout, measuring 20 feet wide by 44 feet long. The court is divided into two halves by a net that stands 36 inches high at the sidelines and 34 inches high at the center. On either side of the net, there are two service courts and a 7-foot Non-Volley Zone, commonly referred to as "the kitchen," extending from the net.

pickleball doubles: Pickleball doubles is a game format where two teams, each consisting of two players, compete against each other on the pickleball court.

pickleball footwork: Pickleball footwork refers to the movement and positioning of the feet on the court, involving quick steps, pivots, shuffles, and lunges to reach the ball efficiently and maintain balance.

pickleball kit: A pickleball kit is a package or set that includes various items needed to play the sport. It is designed to provide beginners or new players with a convenient way to acquire the essential equipment all at once. A typical pickleball kit may contain

pickleball singles: Pickleball singles is a game format where two players compete against each other on the pickleball court, with one player on each side of the net.

pickleball skill rating: This is a system used to assess and categorize players based on their skill level in the game. It provides a standardized way to measure and communicate a player's proficiency and helps ensure fair competition among players of similar abilities.

pickleball spin: Pickleball spin refers to the various types of spin that can be applied to the ball, including topspin, backspin, sidespin, or combinations of these spins, influencing the ball's trajectory and bounce.

pickleball strategy: Pickleball strategy refers to the game plan or approach that players employ to gain an advantage over their opponents, involving shot selection, court positioning, and tactical decisions.

pickler: A "pickler" refers to an enthusiastic player or fan of pickleball.

poach: Poach refers to a strategic move where a player crosses over into their partner's area of the court to intercept or take a shot intended for their partner, often executed to surprise the opponents and gain an advantage.

power: Power, in the context of pickleball, refers to the force or strength with which a shot is struck. It is the ability to generate speed and energy in the movement of the paddle, resulting in a fast and impactful shot.

Professional Pickleball Association (PPA): A professional organization dedicated to promoting and advancing the sport of pickleball at the highest level. It is one of the major governing bodies for professional pickleball in the United States. The PPA organizes and sanctions professional pickleball tournaments that attract top players from around the world.

punch: To punch in pickleball means to hit the ball with a quick and short stroke, often used for controlled shots or when the ball is closer to the body.

punch volley: A punch volley is a short and quick shot played with a sharp forward motion of the paddle, generating power and speed to place the ball precisely and surprise the opponent.

pure winner: A pure winner is a shot that is hit with such precision and skill that it lands in a position where the opponent has no chance of returning it, resulting in an immediate point or winning shot.

put-away: A put-away refers to a shot or play that finishes the rally by effectively ending the point, often executed with power and placement to prevent the opponent from making a return.

rally: A rally in pickleball refers to a sequence of shots exchanged between players, starting from the serve and continuing until the point is won or lost.

rallying: Where both teams exchange shots, aiming to keep the ball in play.

rally scoring system: This is a scoring method where points are awarded on every rally, regardless of which team serves, adding a fast-paced and competitive element to the game.

receiver: The receiver is the player who receives the serve from the opposing team and initiates the rally.

ready position: The stance and posture adopted by a player in anticipation of the opponent's shot, with knees slightly bent, weight balanced, and paddle prepared for quick reaction and movement.

referee: A referee is an official responsible for ensuring fair play, enforcing the rules, and making judgments or decisions during pickleball matches or tournaments.

reset: To reset in pickleball means to regain control or neutralize the rally by hitting a safe shot that returns the ball over the net without taking excessive risks.

resetting: The act of returning the ball to a neutral position during transition play.

return of serve: This refers to the shot played by the receiving player or team in response to the opponent's serve. It is the first stroke executed after the serve and marks the beginning of a rally.

right/even service box: The right service box, also known as the even service box, is the service box on the right-hand side of the court as viewed from the serving team's perspective.

round robin: Round robin is a tournament format where participants compete against every other player or team in the tournament, ensuring that each player has a chance to play against all other players in their category or group.

score: The score in pickleball refers to the numerical representation of points earned by each team or player during a game or match, determining the progress and outcome of the competition.

second server: The second server comes into play when the first server commits a fault by serving out of bounds or into the net. In such cases, the second server from the serving team takes over the serving duty and serves from the same service position as the first server. The second server continues serving until they commit a fault, at which point the serve would rotate to the opposing team, or until their team wins the point and retains the serve.

serve: The serve in pickleball is the action of initiating play by striking the ball from behind the baseline and into the opponent's service box, commencing the rally.

serve number: Serve number refers to the order or position in which players take turns serving in a game or match. In doubles pickleball, the score is made up of three numbers (for instance, 0-0-2). The first number represents the serving team's score. The second number represents the receiving team's score. The third number represents the server number, which is either server #1 or server #2.

serve outside scoring: Serve outside scoring is a scoring system used in some variations of pickleball where only the serving team can score points. In this system, if the receiving team wins a rally, they do not score a point. Instead, they gain the opportunity to serve. This means that only the serving team can accumulate points during their own service turn.

server: The server is the player who executes the serve to start the rally and initiates play from behind the baseline.

server number: The server number refers to the position or order in which players take turns serving in a game or match. In doubles pickleball, the score is made up of three numbers (for instance, 0-0-2). The first number represents the serving team's score. The second number represents the receiving team's score. The third number represents the server number, which is either server #1 or server #2

service box: The service box is a rectangular area on each side of the net where the server must stand and serve the ball into the opponent's service box to begin the rally.

service court: The terms "service court" and "service box" are often used interchangeably in pickleball. Both refer to the area on either side of the net where the ball must land when served.

serving team: This is the team that begins the rally by serving the ball over the net to the opposing team. They have the responsibility of initiating the game and scoring points. The serving team rotates their serving position after each point is won.

setup: A setup in pickleball refers to a shot or situation that provides an advantageous opportunity for the player to execute a winning shot or put-away.

Shake 'N' Bake: Shake 'N' Bake is a term used to describe a play where the serving team follows up the serve with an aggressive and quick volley or shot, putting pressure on the opponent and aiming to win the point.

short serve: A short serve in pickleball is a serve that lands closer to the Non-Volley Zone or kitchen line on the receiving side. It is the opposite of the deep serve.

shot: Refers to the specific technique or action used to hit the ball during gameplay, such as the lob, drive, dink, or drop shot, with the aim of achieving a desired outcome and strategically challenging opponents.

shot selection: The strategic process of choosing and executing a specific type of shot in pickleball based on factors such as ball trajectory, opponent position, court positioning, and desired outcome.

sideline: The sideline refers to the boundary line running along the length of the pickleball court, marking the outer edge and determining whether a shot or ball is considered in or out of bounds.

side out: A side out occurs when the serving team loses the rally, resulting in the serve switching to the opposing team.

sidespin: Sidespin is a type of spin applied to the ball in pickleball, causing it to rotate horizontally, resulting in curved trajectories and altering the bounce and movement of the ball.

sideways shuffle: This refers to a lateral movement technique used to quickly and efficiently cover the court laterally. It involves shuffling the feet in a sideways direction while maintaining a low and balanced stance. The sideways shuffle is commonly used to defend against wide shots, move laterally to cover the Non-Volley Zone, or position oneself for an offensive shot.

singles: Singles is a game format in pickleball where two players compete against each other on the court, with one player on each side of the net.

sitter: A sitter refers to an easy or straightforward shot that is within reach and provides an excellent opportunity for the player to execute a winning shot or put-away.

skinny singles: Skinny singles refers to a game format in pickleball where the width of the court is reduced, creating narrower alleys on each side, making the court more challenging to cover and requiring precise shot placement.

slammer: A slammer in pickleball refers to a powerful and aggressive shot played with force and speed, aimed at overwhelming the opponent and ending the rally.

slice: A slice is a shot played with underspin, where the paddle strikes the bottom of the ball, causing it to rotate backward and create a low, skidding trajectory.

smash (overhead smash or overhead shot): A smash, also known as an overhead smash or overhead shot, is a forceful and powerful shot played from above the player's head with the intention of hitting the ball down with speed and aggression.

soft drop shot: This involves hitting the ball with a gentle touch, causing it to land close to the net and bounce low, making it difficult for your opponent to return.

soft hands: Refers to a player's ability to delicately and accurately control the ball with a gentle touch. It involves applying the right amount of force to execute precise shots, such as dinks and drop shots, while maintaining control and feel. Developing soft hands is crucial for mastering the subtleties of pickleball and enhancing shot-making skills.

specific muscle activation (exercises): Exercises that target the muscles used in pickleball and help activate them before the game. These exercises engage the major muscle groups, improve joint mobility, and enhance readiness for action.

spin: This refers to the rotational movement imparted on the ball when it is struck. It alters the ball's trajectory, speed, and bounce

split step: A split step is a technique used by players to maintain balance and react quickly by jumping or springing into the air just before their opponent makes contact with the ball.

stacking: Stacking is a strategy employed in doubles play where players arrange themselves in a specific formation on the same side of the court, typically to gain a better angle for their shots or exploit their strengths.

stance: Refers to the posture or position of the body assumed by a player in preparation for engaging in an activity or sport. In pickleball, the stance refers to the specific positioning of the feet, legs, and body that provides a stable and balanced foundation for executing shots, moving on the court, and reacting to the game.

starting over: Starting over refers to the process of resetting or returning to the initial score or game state, often occurring in situations where the game or match needs to be replayed due to a specific circumstance or interruption.

starting server: The starting server in pickleball is the player who serves first at the beginning of the game, determined by a coin toss or rally.

strategic ventilation: Strategic ventilation in pickleball clothing refers to the incorporation of breathable materials, such as mesh or perforated panels, in areas that tend to get hot and sweaty during gameplay. It allows for better airflow, helps regulate body temperature, and enhances overall comfort and performance on the court.

stretches: Specific exercises or movements that aim to elongate and loosen the muscles and tendons in the body. These stretching exercises are performed before and after playing pickleball to improve flexibility, increase range of motion, and prevent muscle tightness and injury.

stroke: A stroke in pickleball refers to the specific technique used to hit the ball with the paddle, including shots such as groundstrokes, volleys, serves, and other types of paddle contact with the ball.

sweet spot: The sweet spot refers to the specific area on the paddle's surface that provides the optimal combination of power, control, and accuracy when hitting the ball. Hitting the ball on the sweet spot results in a cleaner and more efficient shot, maximizing the player's performance. Typically located near the center of the paddle, the sweet spot is the desired target for players to consistently aim for during gameplay.

swinging volley: A swinging volley is a shot played with a full swing while the ball is in the air, usually executed closer to the net, allowing the player to hit the ball aggressively and maintain control of the rally.

tagging: Tagging in pickleball refers to the action of touching or tagging the Non-Volley Zone or kitchen line with any part of the player's body or equipment, resulting in a fault.

third shot: The third shot refers to the shot that the serving team hits after their opponent returns the serve, often played with the aim of positioning themselves into a more advantageous position on the court.

third shot drop: The third shot drop in pickleball refers to a shot played by the serving team as their third shot, typically a soft and controlled shot that lands close to the net in the opponent's Non-Volley Zone.

three-quarters stack: The three-quarters stack is a doubles positioning strategy where one player stands closer to the middle of the court, slightly behind the Non-Volley Zone, while their partner stands further back on the same side.

tiebreak: A tiebreak in pickleball is a method used to determine the winner of a game when the score is tied. The specific rules for a tiebreak can vary depending on the tournament or league, but generally, a tiebreak involves playing additional points until one player or team reaches a certain number of points and wins by a margin of at least two points.

time-out: A time-out is a pause or break in play, often called by a team or player to regroup, discuss strategy, or disrupt the momentum of the opposing team.

topspin: Topspin is a type of spin applied to the ball in pickleball, causing it to rotate forward, resulting in a higher bounce and a more aggressive trajectory.

tournament: A tournament is a structured competition where players or teams compete against each other in a series of matches or games, aiming to achieve the highest ranking or win the championship.

traditional/standard/volley serve: The traditional, standard, or volley serve in pickleball refers to a serve where you toss or drop the ball and hit it before it bounces. The ball needs to be hit below your waist height, and in an upwards arc. This type of serve used to be the only serve allowable until the drop serve became a provisional rule in 2021.

traditional or side-out scoring system: The traditional or side-out scoring system in pickleball is a method where only the serving team can score points. The serving team must win the rally to earn a point, while the receiving team's goal is to regain the serve. The serving team continues to serve until they commit a fault, at which point the serve goes to the opposing team. The first team to reach a specified number of points with a minimum lead of two points wins the game.

trajectory: Trajectory refers to the path or flight pattern that an object follows as it moves through space. It specifically refers to the path of the ball after it is struck by a player's paddle and describes the direction and arc the ball takes as it travels towards the opponent's court.

transition: Transition in pickleball refers to the movement and adjustment made by players as they transition from a defensive position to an offensive position or vice versa during a rally. This can involve moving closer to or further away from the net, adjusting the position of the paddle, or changing the type of shot being played.

transition area: The transition area, often referred to as the "no man's land," is the region between the Non-Volley Zone and the baseline.

transition zone: The transition zone is the area on the pickleball court between the Non-Volley Zone and the baseline, where players often find themselves moving and adjusting their position during rallies.

tweener: A tweener is a shot played between the legs or with an unconventional technique, often used as a last resort to reach and return a ball that is challenging to reach in a traditional manner.

two and out: Two and out refers to a scenario where a team loses a rally immediately after serving twice in a row, resulting in the loss of the serve and a side out.

two-bounce rule: The two-bounce rule in pickleball states that after the serve, both teams must let the ball bounce once on each side of the net before volleys are allowed, ensuring fair play and longer rallies.

two-handed backhand: The two-handed backhand in pickleball refers to a backhand shot or stroke where the player grips the paddle with both hands, providing increased stability and power.

unattackable ball: An unattackable ball refers to a shot or ball that is placed in a way that makes it challenging for the opponent to execute an offensive shot in response, often resulting in a defensive or neutral return.

underhand serve: This is a type of serve where the player strikes the ball with an underhand motion, swinging their arm upward from below their waist to make contact with the ball. Unlike an overhand serve, which involves a throwing motion, the underhand serve is performed with a swinging motion below the waist.

underspin or **backspin**: Underspin or backspin is a type of spin applied to the ball in pickleball, causing it to rotate backward, resulting in a lower bounce and slower speed.

unforced error: An unforced error refers to a mistake or error made by a player that is not caused by pressure or an opponent's shot, often resulting in the loss of a point due to a self-inflicted error.

upper-body mechanics: Refers to the movements and actions performed by the upper body, including the arms, shoulders, and torso, during pickleball. It encompasses techniques and motions involved in striking the ball, such as the swing, follow-through, and coordination of the upper body to generate power, control, and accuracy in shots.

USA Pickleball: USA Pickleball is the national governing body for the sport of pickleball in the United States. It was formerly known as the USA Pickleball Association. The organization is responsible for promoting the growth and development of pickleball, maintaining the official rules of the game, sanctioning tournaments, and providing player ratings. USA Pickleball also offers resources and support to players, coaches, and officials.

UPTPR (USAPA Tournament Player Rating): UPTPR, or USAPA Tournament Player Rating, is a rating system used by the USA Pickleball Association to assess the skill level of tournament players based on their performance and results.

volley: A volley in pickleball is a shot played in the air without the ball bouncing, typically executed close to the net, often requiring quick reflexes and control to hit the ball before it touches the ground.

warm-ups: Essential pre-exercise routines designed to prepare the body for physical activity.

weak side: In pickleball, the weak side of a player refers to their weaker shot, which is often their backhand side. Most pickleball players have stronger forehand shots than backhand shots. A common strategy on the pickleball court is to find your opponents' weakness and target that weakness.

western grip: The western grip is a pickleball grip where the hand is positioned further to the right side of the paddle (for right-handed players), with the index knuckle moving closer to the center of the paddle face. This grip allows for more power and topspin on shots, but it can limit maneuverability and control.

windscreen: A windscreen in pickleball refers to a barrier or fence installed around the court, often made of fabric or mesh, to reduce the impact of wind on the game and improve visibility.

wood: Pickleball paddles are commonly made using a variety of wood types, such as plywood, hardwood, or composite wood materials. The specific type of wood used can vary depending on the manufacturer and the desired characteristics of the paddle, including its weight, durability, and playing performance.

Made in the USA
Las Vegas, NV
16 August 2023

76157509R00113